Healthcare Management (Second Edition)

OrangeBooks Publication

Smriti Nagar, Bhilai, Chhattisgarh - 490020

Website:**www.orangebooks.in**

Second Edition, 2023

First Edition, 2021

2ND EDITION (WITH MCQs)

HEALTHCARE MANAGEMENT

ANAM FARUQI

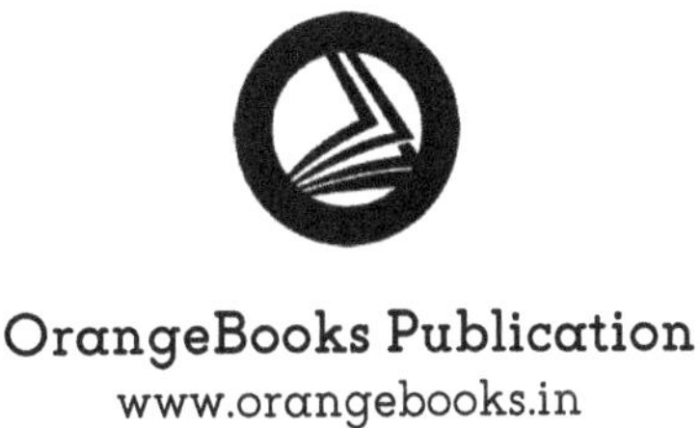

OrangeBooks Publication
www.orangebooks.in

Dedicated to
My Mum
Prof. Roshan Ara
&
My Daddy
Prof. Nafis Ahmad Faruqi

Preface to the Second Edition

The First Edition of this book has evoked positive and encouraging response from the readers. A State University has included it as 'text book' in the syllabus of a Post Graduate course in Hospital Management. It is also recommended for the State Public Service Commission Hospital Care Taker Exam.

In the Second Edition, the first chapter is rewritten to incorporate current data in it. Some minor editing is also done in other chapters to keep them up to date and free from typing errors. Multiple Choice Questions are added at the end of each chapter. They would help readers to assess their knowledge and understanding of the subject.

This book is intended for students pursuing hospital management courses as well as those appearing for competitive exams.

I am extremely thankful to the entire team of OrangeBooks Publication for bringing out the Second Edition of this book.

Anam Faruqi

Preface to the First Edition

An analysis of healthcare system is done to understand its functioning and to suggest ways to improve its performance. Healthcare strategy provides a framework for making day to day choices in alignment with objectives of an organization. Nowadays, healthcare has emerged as a key component of service sector with main focus on quality. The quality of healthcare is measured by its effectiveness and efficiency. Healthcare organizations take initiatives to promote safety. Regulation and accreditation play an important role in ensuring patient safety and quality of care. Health information technology has the potential to improve patient safety by reducing medication errors and improving compliance to practice guidelines. Healthcare needs to be accessible and affordable to all. Telemedicine is one such application that aims to achieve this goal. Improving patient care has become a priority for healthcare providers with the overall objective of achieving high degree of patient satisfaction.

This book is divided into six chapters. The first chapter 'Analytical Study of Healthcare Systems' analyzes different healthcare systems around the world and discusses their merits and demerits. The second chapter 'Strategic Perspectives of Healthcare Leadership' throws light on the role of strategic planning in healthcare and gives an insight into the strategic framework of Indian healthcare market. The third chapter 'Quality and Safety Issues in Healthcare Facility' points out the relevance of quality and safety in the delivery of healthcare. The fourth chapter 'Role of Informatics in Healthcare Delivery' explores different applications of informatics in healthcare. The fifth chapter 'Telemedicine: An Emerging Trend in Healthcare Technology' examines the contribution of public and private sector in promoting treatment through telemedicine in India. The sixth chapter 'Importance of Patience Experience in Healthcare Planning' stresses on the significance of patient experience in providing healthcare.

This book is intended for the students pursuing hospital management courses as well as healthcare industry professionals.

A lucid style of writing has been adopted throughout this book and sincere effort has been made to keep it free from typing errors.

Anam Faruqi

Contents

Chapter 2

Chapter 3

Chapter 4

Role of Informatics in Healthcare Delivery **87**

Chapter 5

Telemedicine: An Emerging Trend in Healthcare Technology **110**

Chapter 6

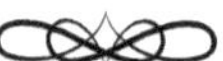

Chapter 1

Analytical Study of Healthcare Systems

Abstract

There is a great disparity in terms of services provided by healthcare systems worldwide. Developed countries score much better on health parameters like life expectancy, cancer survival rates, incidence of chronic diseases etc. On the other hand, developing nations struggle to provide basic healthcare facilities to their citizens. This chapter analyzes healthcare systems of both developed and developing nations, highlights their pros and cons and suggests ways to improve so that affordable quality care is provided to all without any discrimination.

Introduction

Healthcare leaders and professionals need to have a broad understanding of a variety of healthcare systems that exist across the globe. One should be exposed to different types of healthcare delivery systems in order to incorporate innovations in one's organization.

Let's have a look at different healthcare systems around the globe.

United States Healthcare System

The United States Department of Health and Human Services (HHS) is a branch of the federal government that provides governance over healthcare services.

Following are some of the important agencies that HHS governs-

(a) Centers for Medicare and Medicaid Services (CMS)

It is a federal program that provides healthcare services to a variety of consumers. Medicare provides health services to adults of the age of 65 years or older and individuals with documented disabilities. Medicaid and the Children's Health Insurance Plan (CHIP) combine federal resources along with state governments to provide healthcare services to low income population.

(b) Centers for Disease Control and Prevention (CDC)

It conducts research and programs to protect health and safety.

(c) National Institute of Health (NIH)

It is responsible for biomedical and health related research.

(d) Health Resources and Services Administration (HRSA)

It supports the efforts to improve healthcare access for people that are uninsured, isolated or medically vulnerable.

(e) Agency for Healthcare Research and Quality (AHRQ)

It conducts evidence based research on practices, outcomes, effectiveness, clinical guidelines, safety, patient experience, health information technology and health disparities.

(f) Food and Drug Administration (FDA)

It is responsible for promoting public health through regulation of food, tobacco products, pharmaceutical drugs, medical devices and vaccines etc.

Affordable Care Act

In 2010, government of the United States passed the Affordable Care Act which established a shared responsibility for healthcare, between the government, employers and individuals. This plan was designed to provide affordable and quality healthcare to the citizens of the U.S.

Affordable Care Act covers ten essential health benefit categories namely ambulatory patient services, emergency services, hospitalization, maternity and newborn care, mental health services and substance use disorder treatment, prescription drugs, rehabilitative services and devices, laboratory services, preventive and wellness services and chronic disease management and pediatric services including dental and vision care.

The Affordable Care Act resulted in an estimated 20 million gaining coverage, reducing the share of uninsured adults aged 19 to 64 from 20% in 2010 to 12% in 2018.

The United States has no single nationwide system of health insurance. Health insurance is purchased in the private market place or provided by the government to certain groups.

In 2018, about 67% of the U.S. population is covered by private voluntary health insurance (55% received employer provided insurance and 11% acquired coverage directly) and 34% is covered by public health insurance (Medicare, Medicaid, CHIP and military). In 2018, 8.5% of the U.S. population is estimated to lack health insurance coverage. This does not mean these individuals are without access to healthcare services. Many uninsured people receive healthcare services through public clinics and hospitals. State and local health programs or private providers finance the care through charity and by shifting costs to other payers.

Primary care physicians account for about one third of all the U.S. doctors. Patients generally have free choice of doctor, and are usually not required to register with a primary care practice, depending on their insurance plan. Physicians are paid through a combination of methods like negotiated fees (private insurance), capitation (private insurance and some public insurance) and administratively set fees (public insurance).

Specialists can work in both private practice and hospitals. Some insurance plans require a referral by a primary care doctor to see a specialist while others allow direct access. Specialists are paid through the same way as that of primary care physicians.

In 2018, 57% of the 5,198 short term acute care hospitals in the U.S. were non profit, 25% were for profit and 19% were public (state or local government owned). In addition there were 209 federal government hospitals. Hospitals are paid through a combination of methods, including per service, or per diem charges, per case payments and bundled payments, in which case the hospital may be financially accountable for readmissions and services rendered by other providers following discharge.

Mental health care is provided by a mix of for profit and non-profit providers and professionals including primary care physicians, psychiatrists, psychologists, social workers and nurses. They are paid through a range of methods depending upon the provider type and payer. Many insurance plans cover patient hospitalization, outpatient treatment, emergency care , prescription drugs etc.

German Healthcare System

Health insurance is mandatory for all citizens and permanent residents of Germany.

It is provided by two systems-

1. Statutory Health Insurance (SHI)

2. Private Health Insurance (PHI)

As of 2019, all employed citizens (and other groups such as pensioners) earning less than EUR 60,750 (USD 77,985) per year are mandatorily covered by SHI, and their non-earning dependents are covered free of charge. Individuals whose gross wages exceed the threshold and the previously SHI insured self employed can remain in the publicly financed scheme on a voluntary basis (as 75% do) or purchase substitutive PHI, which also covers civil servants.

About 88% of the population receives their primary coverage through SHI and 11% through substitutive PHI. Military members, police and other public sector employees are covered under special programs.

Statutory Health Insurance covers preventive services, inpatient and outpatient hospital care, physician services, mental health care, dental care, optometry, physical therapy, prescription drugs, medical aids, rehabilitation, hospice and palliative care and sick leave compensation. Preventive services under SHI include regular dental checkups, child checkups, basic immunization, checkups for chronic diseases and cancer screening at certain ages.

In 2017, family physicians, including GPs, internists and pediatricians, accounted for 45% of self employed, SHI contracted ambulatory care physicians (57,600 of roughly 1,29,000), while 55% (71,400) were specialists.

Individuals have free choice among GPs, specialists and if referred to inpatient care, hospitals.

Public hospitals make up about half of all beds, while private non-for profit account for about a third. The total number of private, for profit hospitals has been growing in recent years (now accounting for about one sixth of all beds).

Acute psychiatric inpatient care is largely provided by psychiatric wards in general (acute) hospitals.

Canadian Healthcare System

In Canada, there is 100% insurance coverage through Medicare, funded and administered primarily by provinces and territories. Also, 67% of the Canadian population is covered by private complementary insurance.

Provincial and territorial insurance plans cover physician, diagnostic and hospital services (including inpatient prescription drugs) for all eligible residents. They also provide varying levels of additional benefits such as outpatient prescription drugs, non physician mental health care, vision care, dental care, home care and hospice care.

Provincial and territorial government's insurance plans also provide public health and prevention services (including immunization) as part of their public programs.

In 2017, there were 2.3 practicing physicians per 1000 population, about half of whom were general practitioners (1.2 per 1000 population) and the rest specialists (1.15 per 1000 population).

Patients have free choice of primary care doctor.

The majority of specialist care is provided in hospitals. Patients can choose and have direct access to a specialist, but it is common for general physicians to refer patients to specialty care.

Hospitals are a mix of public and private. There is a universal coverage for physician provided mental health care.

Swiss Healthcare System

In the Swiss healthcare system, duties and responsibilities are divided among the federal, cantonal and municipal levels of government. Each of the 26 cantons has its own constitution and is responsible for licensing healthcare providers, coordinating hospital services and subsidizing institutions and individual premiums. The federal government plays an important role in regulating the financing of the system. Municipalities are responsible mainly for long term care and other social support services for vulnerable groups.

In Switzerland, Mandatory Health Insurance (MHI) is universal. Residents are legally required to purchase it within three months of their arrival in Switzerland. Mandatory Health Insurance covers most general practitioner and specialist services as well as pharmaceuticals and medical devices, home care services, maternity care, physiotherapy and some preventive measures including the cost of selected vaccination and screening for early detection of diseases among certain risk groups.

Hospital services are also covered by Mandatory Health Insurance. Care for mental illness is covered if it is provided by certified physicians.

Dental care is excluded. Glasses and contact lenses for adults are excluded but it is included for children under 18.

In Switzerland, registering with a GP is not required, so people have free choice among self employed GPs. In 2017, 42.9% of doctors in the outpatient sector were classified as GPs, while 57.1% were classified as specialists.

In 2016, there were 283 hospitals (102 general and 181 specialty hospitals) with a total of 38,058 beds.

Norwegian Healthcare System

Norway has universal health and social insurance coverage known as the National Insurance Scheme (NIS).

The Norwegian government is responsible for providing healthcare to the population with equal access to care regardless of age, race, gender, income or area of residency. Providing primary health and social care is the responsibility of the municipalities with Norway's ministry of health playing an indirect role through legislation and funding mechanisms. In specialist care, the ministry plays a direct role through its ownership of hospitals and its provision of directives to the boards of regional healthcare authorities.

National healthcare covers planned and acute primary health services, hospital stays, ambulatory care, mental health treatment, rehabilitation, outpatient prescription medicines, preventive services and maternity care. It also covers dental care for children up to 18 years of age and people with chronic medical diseases.

About 10% of the Norwegian population is covered by private supplementary insurance. It gives quicker access to elective services and greater choice of private specialists.

In Norway, there is a 'Regular GP Scheme' whereby people register with one primary general practitioner. A GP referral is required for coverage of specialist treatment.

There are 2.8 specialists in hospitals or ambulatory care for every practicing primary care physician.

Public hospitals are state owned and are governed by an executive board. There are few private hospitals that are generally owned by humanitarian organizations.

Mental health services are funded 100% by grants.

Chinese Healthcare System

Chinese healthcare system is based on the principle that every person has a basic right to healthcare services.

In China, the central government is overall responsible for national health legislation, policy and administration.

In China, coverage by publicly financed health insurance is near universal.

Publicly financed insurance covers primary, specialist, emergency department, hospital and mental health care, physical therapy as well as prescription drugs and traditional medicines. Preventive services such as immunization and disease screening are included in a separate public health benefit package funded by central and local governments.

Primary care is delivered mainly through village doctors and health workers in rural clinics, general practitioners in rural township and urban community hospitals and medical professionals in secondary and tertiary hospitals. Village doctors are not licensed GPs and are only able to provide care in rural areas.

In 2018, there were 9,07,098 village doctors and health workers providing care in rural areas. Patients can see a specialist without a referral from a G.P. and can choose a specialist through the hospital. In 2018, China had 3,08,740 licensed and assistant GPs.

In China, hospitals can be private, non-profit or for profit. In 2018, there were approximately 12,000 public hospitals and 21,000 private hospitals. There were 5,06,003 public primary care facilities and 4,37,636 private village clinics that provide care to residents.

Mental care is provided by specialty psychiatric hospitals and clinics.

Australian Healthcare System

Australia has universal public health insurance program known as Medicare.

In Australia, the federal, state and local governments are collectively responsible for providing universal healthcare. The federal government mainly provides funding and indirect support to the states, subsidizing primary care providers through Medicare Benefits Scheme (MBS) and Pharmaceutical Benefits Scheme (PBS) and providing funds for state services.

Medicare Benefits Scheme (MBS) includes hospital care, medical services etc.

Pharmaceutical Benefits Scheme (PBS) provides pharmaceutical subsidies.

States have the major responsibility for public hospitals, ambulance services, public dental care, community health services and mental health care. They contribute their own funding in addition to that provided by federal government.

Local governments play a role in the delivery of community health and preventive health programs such as immunization and the regulation of food standards.

Nearly half of the Australian population (46%) has private supplementary coverage. It offers more choice of providers (particularly in hospitals), faster access to non-emergency services and rebates for selected services.

In 2015, there were 34,367 general physicians and 8,386 specialists.

Registration with a GP is not required and patients can choose their primary care doctor.

Specialists deliver outpatient care in private practice or in a public hospital. Patients are able to choose their own specialist but must be referred by their GP to receive MBS subsidies.

In 2016-17, there were 695 public hospitals with a total of nearly 60,300 beds. There were 630 private hospitals with 33,100 beds. Private hospitals are a mix of for profit and non-profit.

Public hospitals receive a majority of funding (92%) from the federal government and state governments.

Mental health services are provided by GPs and specialists.

French Healthcare System

In France, providing health care is the national responsibility. Responsibilities of the central government include setting national health strategy, allocating budgeted expenditures among different sectors (hospitals, ambulatory care, mental health and services for disabled residents) and regions.

The Ministry is represented in regions by the regional health agencies which are responsible for coordinating population health and healthcare, including prevention and care delivery, public health and social health.

Health and social care for elderly and disabled people come under the jurisdiction of General Councils which are governing bodies at the local level.

In French healthcare system, coverage is universal and compulsory, provided to all residents by non-competitive Statutory Health Insurance (SHI).

SHI covers hospital care and treatment in public or private rehabilitation or physiotherapy institutions; outpatient care provided by general practitioners, specialists, dentists and midwives; all maternity care services, from the 12th week of pregnancy to six months after delivery; newborn care and children's preventive health care up to age 4; diagnostic services prescribed by doctors and carried out by laboratories and paramedical professionals; prescription drugs, medical appliances and prostheses that have been approved for reimbursement and prescribed healthcare related transportation and home care. It also partially covers long term hospice and mental health care and provides only minimal coverage to outpatient vision and dental care. While preventive services in general receive limited coverage, there is a full reimbursement for targeted services such as immunization, mammography and colorectal cancer screening as well as for preventive care for targeted population.

Also, 95% of the French population is covered by private complementary insurance.

There are roughly 1,02,299 general practitioners (GPs) and 1,21,272 specialists in France.

Patients can choose among specialists upon referral by a GP with the exception of gynaecologists, ophthalmologists, psychiatrists and stomatologists. Bypassing referral results in reduced SHI coverage.

In France, public institutions account for about 65% of hospital capacity and activity, private for profit facilities account for another 25% and private non-profit facilities, the main providers of cancer treatment, make up the remainder.

Services for mentally ill people are provided by both public and private healthcare sectors.

New Zealand Healthcare System

In New Zealand, the government has a central role in providing population's healthcare needs. Responsibility for planning, purchasing and providing health services as well as disability support for those over age 65, lies on 20 geographically defined District Health Boards (DHBs), each of which comprises seven locally elected members and up to four members appointed by the Ministry of Health. These boards pursue government objectives, targets and service requirements while operating government owned hospitals and health centers, providing community services and purchasing services from non government and private providers.

Publicly funded insurance system covers preventive care; inpatient and outpatient hospital services; primary care via private providers (excluding services such as optometry, adult dental services, orthodontics and physiotherapy); maternity services; physical therapy; durable medical equipment; inpatient and outpatient prescription drugs; mental health care; dental care for school children; long term care; homecare; hospice care and disability support services.

Private complementary insurance covers 33% of the New Zealand's population. It is used mostly to cover cost sharing requirements, elective surgery in private hospitals and private outpatient specialist consultations.

In New Zealand, the ratio of GPs to specialists is about 2:3. There is a mix of public and private hospitals but public hospitals constitute the majority providing all emergency and intensive care.

Most people get access to mental health care through community based primary mental health services, often through their GP, who will then coordinate any referred services.

Dutch Healthcare System

In Netherlands, the national government is overall responsible for setting healthcare priorities, introducing legislative changes whenever needed and monitoring access, quality and costs. It also partly finances social health insurance (a comprehensive system with universal coverage) for the basic benefit package and the compulsory social health insurance system for long term care. Municipalities and health insurers are responsible for most outpatient long term services.

Health insurers are legally required to provide a standard benefits package that includes care provided by general practitioners (GPs), hospitals and specialists; maternal care; dental care up to age 18; prescription drugs; physiotherapy up to age 18; home nursing care; a limited number of health promotion programs, including those for smoking cessation and some weight management advice; basic ambulatory mental health care for mild to moderate mental disorders; and specialized outpatient and inpatient mental care for complicated and severe mental disorders.

In 2017, there were 13,364 registered primary care doctors (GPs) and 23,236 medical specialists.

In 2018, there were 71 hospital organizations, including eight university medical centers. All hospitals are private entities, but profits may not be distributed to shareholders, making the hospital market virtually 100% non profit.

Swedish Healthcare System

All three levels of Swedish government are involved in the healthcare system. At the national level, the Ministry of Health and Social Affairs is responsible for healthcare policy, working in concert with eight national government agencies. At the regional level, 21 regional bodies are responsible for financing and delivering health services to the citizens. At the local level, 290 municipalities are responsible for care of elderly and disabled. Local and regional authorities are represented by the Swedish Association of Local Authorities and Regions (SALAR).

In Sweden, health insurance is publicly financed, universal and automatic. It covers public health and preventive services; primary care, including maternity care; inpatient and outpatient specialized care; emergency care; inpatient and outpatient prescription drugs; mental health care; rehabilitation services, including physical therapy; disability support services, including durable medical equipment such as wheelchairs and hearing aids; patient transport support services; home care and long term care, including nursing home care and hospice care; dental care and optometry for children and young people; and adult dental care with limited subsidies.

In Sweden, there are, on an average four to five GPs in a primary care practice. There are about 1,200 primary care practices of which 60% are owned by regions and 40% are privately owned.

Outpatient specialist care is provided at university and regional hospitals and in private clinics.

There are seven university hospitals, all public, and about 70 public community hospitals owned by the regions. There are also six private hospitals, of which three are not for profit.

People with minor mental health problems are usually attended in primary care settings either by a GP or by a psychologist; patients with severe mental health problems are referred to specialized psychiatric care in hospitals.

English Healthcare System

Health coverage in the United Kingdom is universal. Approximately 10.5% of the U.K.'s population also has private voluntary health insurance.National Health Service (NHS) is the publicly funded healthcare system in England and one of the four National Health Service Systems in the United Kingdom.

NHS provides healthcare to all legal English residents and residents from other regions of the United Kingdom. NHS provides or pays for preventive services, including screening, immunization and vaccination programs; inpatient and outpatient hospital care; maternity care; physician services; inpatient and outpatient drugs; clinically necessary dental care; some eye care; mental health care, including some care for those with learning disabilities; palliative care; some long term care; rehabilitation, including physiotherapy (such as after stroke care); home visits by community based nurses; wheelchairs, hearing aids and other assistive devices.

Primary care is delivered mainly through general practitioners.

In 2017, there were 34,000 general practitioners and 45,800 hospital specialists.

Most GPs (59.4%) are self employed while nearly all specialists are salaried employees of NHS hospitals.

Publicly owned hospitals are organized either as NHS trusts (currently 64) directly accountable to the Department of Health or as foundation trusts (currently 142) regulated by NHS Improvement.

There are about 515 private hospitals.

Mental health care is an integral part of the NHS and covers a full range of services.

Indian Healthcare System

According to the Constitution of India, each State is required to provide free universal access to healthcare services. In practice, however, the private sector is responsible for the majority of healthcare, and most healthcare expenses are paid directly out of pocket by patients and their families, rather than through healthcare insurance. The central government is responsible for international health treaties, medical education, prevention of food adulteration, quality control in drug manufacturing, national disease control and family planning programs.

Government health services are available to all citizens under the tax financed public system.

In 2018, the Central government launched tax financed National Health Protection Scheme (Ayushman Bharat Pradhan Mantri Jan Arogya Yojna or PM-JAY) for low income population. This scheme provides INR 5,00,000 per family per year to cover secondary and tertiary healthcare. This scheme extends coverage to approximately 100 million poor and vulnerable families.

In India, 37% of population is covered by either government or private health insurance scheme.

The government healthcare system is designed as a three tier structure comprising primary, secondary and tertiary facilities. In rural areas, primary healthcare services are provided through a network of sub centers (SCs), primary health centers (PHCs) and community health centers (CHCs).

Sub center is the first point of contact between primary healthcare system and local community, designed to handle maternal and child health, disease control and health counseling for a population of 3000 to 5000. Each sub center is required to be manned by at least one ANM (Auxiliary Nurse Midwife), female health worker and one male health worker. As in 2015, there were 1,52,326 sub centers running in the country.

Primary health center is the first point of contact between village community and medical officer and provides curative and preventive services to 20,000 to 30,000 people. As per the minimum norms, there should be a medical officer supported by 14 paramedical and other staff to manage a PHC. As in 2015, there were 25,020 PHCs functioning in the country. PHC serves as a referral unit for six sub centers and has four to six beds for patients.

Community health centers are managed and maintained by state governments and are required to have four medical specialists supported by 21 paramedical and other staff. They must also have 30 beds, laboratory, x-ray and other facilities. It covers 80,000 to 1,20,000 people.

Secondary healthcare system consists of Sub-Divisional Hospitals (SDHs), District Hospitals (DHs) and Mobile Medical Units (MMUs). As in 2015, there were 1022 SDHs, 763 DHs and 1253 MMUs.

At the tertiary level of healthcare, specialized preventive care is given to the patients usually on referral from primary and secondary healthcare centers. Tertiary healthcare system includes medical colleges and advanced medical research institutes.

Public hospitals account for about 10% of the total number of hospitals throughout the country. The rest are operated by the private for profit sector. There has been significant growth in the number of private sector hospitals because of perceived poor quality care in public facilities and the rise of medical tourism.

With the launch of National Health Protection Scheme, comprehensive mental health care will also be available for beneficiaries at newly established Health and Wellness Centre programs.

Analysis of Healthcare Systems

United States

In healthcare system of the United States, all the citizens are not insured. It is important that more citizens should be covered under Affordable Care Act irrespective of their economic background. The U.S. should strive to provide universal healthcare to its citizens. In the U.S., healthcare spending as a percentage of GDP is 16.9% (highest among all the Nations of the world). It has the highest breast cancer five year net survival rate (90%). The United States healthcare system faces many challenges also. There is relatively high mortality amenable to healthcare (149 deaths per 100,000 population). Obesity rate is also quite high (40%). 28% of the U.S. adults have multiple chronic conditions like arthritis, lung diseases, heart diseases, diabetes, hypertension etc.

Germany

German healthcare system is known for utilization of healthcare resources. Germany has significantly more MRI and CT scanners per capita than other countries (143 per 1000 population). Germany has more doctors and nurses (4.3 and 13.3 per 1000 population respectively) than other developed nations. In Germany, although progress has been made in recent years in reducing unhealthy behavior, smoking (21%) and alcohol consumption (11 liters per year) rates are still above compared to other countries. Obesity rate is also high (23.6%).

Canada

In Canada, the waiting time for healthcare services for specialists and non emergency procedures can be quite long (about 20 weeks). Hospitals can adopt different strategies to deal with it like virtual consultation for primary care etc. Canada spends 10.7% of GDP on healthcare. Canada has 22% adults with multiple chronic conditions. 26.3% Canadians are obese. Canada has high breast cancer five year net survival rate (88%).

Switzerland

In Switzerland, assisted suicide is allowed. In the light of this fact, in the Mandatory Health Insurance, an insurance cover should be provided for the persons who show signs of depression. Government should establish counseling and depression therapy clinics which can treat such patients. In Switzerland, healthcare spending as a percentage of GDP is quite high (12.2%). There is high life expectancy at birth (83.6years). Obesity rate is low (11.3%). Switzerland has high cervical cancer five year net survival rate (71%). There is low mortality amenable to healthcare (90 deaths per 100,000 population).

Norway

In Norway, under the Regular General Practitioner Scheme, all citizens have a right to choose a GP as their regular doctor. This scheme drastically improved patient-doctor stability as well as better GP accessibility. Norway shows promising healthcare outcomes. Cervical cancer five year net survival rate is comparatively high in Norway (73%). Norway has fairly high life expectancy at birth (82.7 years). There is high breast cancer five year net survival rate (88%).

China

In China, rural practitioners play an important role in providing healthcare services. The government should establish training centers for them so that they can provide quality healthcare services.

Australia

In Australia, emergency room waiting time is one of the concerns. At the national level, an average patient has to wait two hours and 48 minutes to receive care. Patients that purchase private health insurance policies can avoid these issues, which is one of the reasons that over half of Australians have private supplementary coverage. Australia has high life expectancy at birth (82.6 years). 30.4% Australians are obese. Australia has pretty high breast cancer five year net survival rate (90%).

France

According to the Euro health consumer index, there is a tendency in the French healthcare system to create a diagnosis for many conditions that need not be medicalized. It means that patients within the system tend to receive more medication that may be unnecessary when compared to other systems of healthcare around the world. France spends 11.2% of GDP on healthcare. France has high life expectancy at birth (82.6 years). There is low mortality amenable to healthcare (90 deaths per 100,000 population). 18% adults in France have multiple chronic conditions.

New Zealand

In New Zealand, one of the major cons of the healthcare system is its exclusivity. There are some criteria that should be met to qualify for public healthcare and if a person is not eligible for public healthcare, he/she will not be able to take out private health insurance either. In New Zealand, life expectancy at birth is 81.9 years. 32.2% of New Zealand's population is obese. New Zealand has high breast cancer five year net survival rate (88%).

Netherlands

In Netherlands, high quality care is provided. Waiting time for the doctor's appointment is comparatively shorter than other countries. Healthcare is quite expensive. In Netherlands, life expectancy at birth is 81.8 years. Netherlands has high breast cancer five year net survival rate (87%).

Sweden

Sweden spends 11% of GDP on healthcare. Sweden has high life expectancy at birth (82.5 years). In Sweden healthcare is widely regarded as of high quality. Sweden has the highest percentage of females aged 50-69 screened for breast cancer (90%). It has high breast cancer five year net survival rate (89%). Cervical cancer five year net survival rate is also considerably high (68%). In Sweden, waiting time to see a doctor can be longer than the patients may prefer. Waiting time to see a specialist can take up to three months.

United Kingdom

In the United Kingdom, life expectancy at birth is 81.3 years. Breast cancer five year net survival rate is 86%. 28.7% of the population is obese. There is high mortality amenable to healthcare (145 deaths per 100,000 population).

India

In India, healthcare spending as a percentage of GDP is 3.6%. A serious drawback of Indian healthcare system is the neglect of rural masses. 70% of India's population lives in rural areas where only 20% of its hospitals are located. It means 80% of hospitals serve 30% of the urban population. Only 34% of the country's doctors serve in rural areas. In India, life expectancy at birth is 70.15 years. According to a study by ASSOCHAM-EY, 40% of the Indian children are undernourished. India has about 77 million diabetics.

Health Disparity

It is the difference in health of a disadvantaged social group and an advantaged social group. Disadvantaged social groups can be poor, racial/ethnic minorities, women, illiterates, disabled etc.

Health Equity

Health equity prioritizes treatment and care based on need. Health professionals, including social workers, community health workers, and public health workers share common responsibility of promoting health equity.

To achieve health equity and improve the overall health of the population, it is necessary to invest more in social determinants of health like education, housing, food security, income supports, employment, maternal and early childhood development and other services that promote health.

Healthcare systems around the world must take initiatives that aim to reduce health disparity and ensure health equity.

Let us look what different healthcare systems have done to reduce health disparities.

United States

In the United States, the Agency for Healthcare Research and Quality publishes an annual national report highlighting disparities in healthcare quality.

Several federal agencies are tasked with monitoring and reducing health disparities.

Their responsibilities include:

(i) Developing policies and programs to eliminate disparities among racial and ethnic minority groups.

(ii) Sanctioning grants to states, local governments and community based organizations for providing care to low income, uninsured or other vulnerable populations.

The Affordable Care Act also has a number of provisions which aim at reducing disparities.

Germany

In Germany, the Health Monitor conducts studies from the patient perspective to assess the performance of the healthcare system. The share of population not satisfied with medical care is very low (0.3%).

Health disparities are implicitly mentioned in the national health targets. A network of more than 120 health related institutions (e.g. sickness funds and their associations) promotes the health of the socially deprived. Sickness funds support 22,000 health related programs.

Canada

In Canada, the Public Health Agency includes health disparities reporting in its mandate and the Canadian Institute for Health Information also reports on disparities in healthcare and health outcomes with a focus on lower income Canadians.

In Ontario, a new strategy to improve the health of indigenous people was launched in 2016, with emphasis on investments in primary care, cultural competency training for healthcare providers, access to fresh fruits and vegetables and mental health services for youth of First Nations.

Switzerland

In Switzerland, health and health access variations are measured and reported publicly by the Swiss Health Survey every five year.

The Swiss Federal Council's National Health 2020 Strategy explicitly calls for improving health opportunities of the most vulnerable population groups such as children, those with low income or with poor educational background, the elderly and immigrants.

Starting in 2018, the National Strategy for the Prevention of Non-Communicable Diseases and the National Strategy on Addiction and Mental Health have focused on health equity.

Norway

In Norway, the Norwegian Institute of Public Health (NIPH) publishes data on social inequality and health. Information about disparities in outcomes and access to care is available through registries and has been studied at the national and regional levels.

The 'Patient and User Rights Act' ensures that all inhabitants have equal access to quality healthcare.

Eliminating socio-economic inequalities in health is a priority of the Directorate for Health. There have been some initiatives for children including vaccination programs and kindergarten and school based programs; initiatives for people with disabilities to be included in the workplace; price and tax policies; initiatives for care integration, general information campaign regarding smoking cessation, alcohol and diet; and specific programs for populations considered at risk.

China

China Health Statistical Yearbook shows that there are still severe disparities in the accessibility and quality of healthcare, although China has made significant improvements in this regard in the past decade.

Disparities in healthcare access are due to variation in insurance benefit packages, urban and rural factors and income inequality. To help bridge the urban-rural healthcare divide, the central government and local governments sponsor training for rural doctors in urban hospitals and require new medical graduates to work as residents in rural health facilities.

Australia

In Australia, the most prominent disparities in health outcomes are between the Aboriginal and Torres Strait Islander population and the rest of Australia's population. Disparities between major urban centers and rural and remote regions and across socio-economic groups are also major challenges. The federal government provides financial incentives to encourage GPs and other health workers to work in rural and remote areas.

This challenge is also addressed to an extent, through the use of telemedicine.

France

In France, reducing disparities with respect to social determinants of health and access to care is a national priority. There is a 6.3 years gap in life expectancy between males in the highest and males in the lowest social categories and poorer self reported health among those with state sponsored insurance and no complementary insurance.

Disparities can be addressed through physician contracts. A contractual agreement allows the use of incentives for physicians practicing in underserved areas, extension of third party payment and enforced limitations on denial of care.

In March 2018, the Minister of Health presented a national plan to reduce health inequalities with a EUR 400 million (USD 506 million) investment over five years and 25 measures that are concerned with all age groups.

New Zealand

In New Zealand, Maori and Pacific Island people have shorter life expectancies than other New Zealanders (by seven and five years respectively) and experience greater difficulty in gaining access to health services. To reduce disparities, many primary health organizations (PHOs) are created especially for Maori and Pacific populations.

Netherlands

In Netherlands, after every four year, variations in health accessibility are measured and published in the Dutch Health Care Performance Reports.

There is a seven years difference in life expectancy between the highest and lowest socio-economic groups. Smoking is still a leading cause of death. In 2013, the government decided to induce diet advice and smoking cessation programs in the statutory benefits package.

Sweden

International comparisons indicate that health disparities are relatively low in Sweden. In Sweden, disparity reduction approaches include programs to support behavioural changes and outpatient preventive programs targeting vulnerable groups.

United Kingdom

In England, National Health Service (NHS) publishes an annual report on the actions taken and progress being made in reducing disparities in healthcare access and outcomes.

NHS strategies include-

(i) Ensuring that local areas receive adequate resources to tackle inequalities.

(ii) Measuring progress towards reducing disparities.

(iii) Providing financial assistance to achieve targeted goals e.g. early detection of cancer.

India

Significant inequalities with respect to healthcare access and outcomes exist between India's states, rural and urban areas, socio-economic groups, castes and genders. For example children in rural areas are about 1.6 times more likely to die before their first birthday and 1.9 times more likely to die before their fifth birthday than those in urban areas. From 1991 to 2013, neonatal mortality declined by 53% in urban areas, compared with 44% in rural areas. The Ministry of Health and Family Welfare strengthened its flagship program, 'National Health Mission' with the aim of reducing health inequalities. Through this program, 9,00,000 accredited social health activists work at the community level to promote immunization, disease control, effective breast feeding and healthy nutrition. Other initiatives seek to reduce maternal mortality e.g. incentivizing women through cash payments to deliver their babies in government health facilities. Recent evidence shows that these policies have reduced disparities in maternal care.

The health inequality can be reduced by providing healthcare services through 'telemedicine' in remote and underserved parts of the nation. In the year 2001, the first telemedicine pilot project was started in India by ISRO (Indian Space Research Organization) in collaboration with Apollo Hospitals Group with the aim of providing affordable healthcare to the rural population.

Health Literacy

Health literacy is a set of skills that people need to function effectively within a healthcare environment.

Following are the types of health literacies-

1. Print literacy

It is the ability to read and understand text, to locate and interpret information in documents, pictures, sign boards etc.

In India, the Ministry of Health and Family Welfare has taken several initiatives to educate people regarding the ill effects of consuming alcohol, tobacco, cigarette etc. One of the initiatives is painting pictures on the public transport depicting the persons having mouth cancer which can be caused by chewing tobacco.

2. Numerical literacy

It is the ability to understand quantitative information. Numerical literacy helps in reading food and beverage labels, measuring blood glucose levels, measuring blood pressure, adhering to a medication management regime etc.

3. Oral literacy

It is the ability to speak and to listen to health information e.g. an individual should be able to understand patient education provided by a health provider like a nurse or a diabetic educator.

Patients with low literacy can face difficulty in:

(i) Filling registration form

(ii) Interacting with physician

(iii) Following medical prescription

(iv) Interpreting food labels

(v) Indulging in self care

Conclusion

It can be concluded that in developed nations, the number of sub specialists has increased at a much higher rate than the number of generalists. This trend leads to fragmented care. To meet the needs of aging population, more family physicians will be needed in future.

Patients suffering from multiple diseases often receive treatment from wide range of providers. Such patients need someone who is responsible for coordinating all their care. In developed countries, healthcare organizations are increasingly employing staff that is specifically tasked with coordinating treatment for complex patient needs. Better coordination leads to better care.

Healthcare providers treating a patient with complex needs should be able to share relevant data about the patient. Electronic record integration can facilitate communication between providers. Patients with complex conditions need to be part of an open discussion about the benefits and risks of individual treatments. Such a process allows bringing their needs, preferences and hopes into the treatment conversation.

Care for mental health must be integrated with physical healthcare, with multidisciplinary teams ensuring that physical and mental problems are addressed together in a timely fashion.

In developing nations like India, preventive care has greater relevance because these countries spend comparatively low on healthcare.

Such countries should adopt preventive care techniques like organizing immunization programs, conducting disease screening, self-checking of blood sugar and blood pressure levels, avoiding consumption of alcohol, tobacco, etc. and maintaining a healthy lifestyle.

Community health workers play an important role in the delivery of primary and preventive care and help in other processes like data collection, conducting immunization programs etc. Community health workers are often members of the communities they serve, so they better understand their needs. In India, where about 70% of the total population lives in rural areas, community health workers help in improving the quality of health of village population.

References

1. Tikkanen, R., & Osborn, R. (Dec, 2020). *International Profiles of Health Care Systems.* The Commonwealth Fund.

2. Berchick, E.R.et al. (Nov, 2019). *Health Insurance Coverage in the United States: 2018 - Current Population Reports.* U.S. Census Bureau.

3. Ridic, G., Gleason, S., & Ridic, O. (June, 2012). Comparisons of Healthcare Systems in the United States, Germany and Canada. *Mat Soc Med, 24(2),* 112-120.

4. Camenzind, P. (2015). The Swiss Health Care System. In E. Mossialos, M. Wenzi, R. Osborn and D. Sarnak (Eds.). *International Profiles of Health Care Systems.* The Commonwealth Fund.

5. *Health at a Glance Europe 2014.* Organization for Economic Co-operation and Development. Nov 19, 2015.

6. Jiang, L., Song, S., & Gno, W. (2014). Study on the Models and Development Status of the Regional Longitudinal Medical Alliance in China. *Medicine and Society, 27(5),* 35-38.

7. *Hospital Resources 2014-15.* Australian Hospital Statistics, Australian Institute of Health and Welfare, Australian Government. 2016.

8. Nay, O., Bejean, S., & Benamouzig, D. et al. (May 28, 2016). Achieving Universal Health Coverage in France: Policy Reforms and the Challenge of Inequalities. *Lancet, 387(10034),* 2236-49.

9. Gauld, R. (Aug 16, 2013). Questions about New Zealand's Health System in 2013, Its 75th Anniversary Year. *New Zealand Medical Journal, 126(1380),* 1-7.

10. Struijs, J.N., & Bann, C.A. (March 17, 2011). Integrating Care through Bundled Payments-Lessons from the Netherlands. *New England Journal of Medicine, 364(11),* 990-91.

11. Anell, A., Glenngard, A. H., & Merkur, S. (2012). Sweden: Health System Review. *Health Systems in Transition, 14(5),* 1-161.

12. *Delivering the Forward View: NHS Planning Guidance 2016/17-2020/21.* NHS England. Dec 2015.

13. Gudwani, A., Mitra, P., & Puri, A., et al. (Jan, 2012). *Indian Healthcare: Inspiring Possibilities, Challenging Journey.* McKinsey and Co.

14. Balarajan, Y., Selvaraj, S., & Subramanian, S .V. (Feb 5, 2011). Health Care and Equity in India. *Lancet, 377(9764),* 505-15.

MCQs

1. Which of the following agencies is not governed by the U.S. Department of Health and Human Services?

a) Centers for Medicare and Medicaid Services

b) National Institute of Health

c) Centers for Disease Control and Prevention

d) National Board for Health Supervision

2. **Which of the following statements is false about the United States Healthcare System?**

   a) The United States has a single nationwide system of health insurance.

   b) Primary care physicians account for about one third of all the U.S. doctors.

   c) Medicare provides health services to adults of the age of 65 years or older and individuals with documented disabilities.

   d) The United States Department of Health and Human Services is a branch of the federal government that provides governance over healthcare services.

3. **In Germany, health insurance is mainly provided by which of the following two systems?**

   a) Medicare Benefits Scheme and Pharmaceutical Benefits Scheme

   b) Statutory Health Insurance and Private Health Insurance

   c) National Insurance Scheme and Private Health Insurance

   d) Medicare and Private Health Insurance

4. **Which of the following statements is true about Canadian Healthcare System?**

   a) There is 100% insurance coverage through Medicare.

   b) 10% of the Canadian population is covered by private complementary insurance.

   c) Physician provided mental health care is excluded in Medicare.

   d) All of the above

5. **Which of the following statements is false about Switzerland's Mandatory Health Insurance?**

   a) It is universal.

   b) It includes dental care for adults.

   c) It covers hospital services.

   d) Residents are legally required to purchase it within three months of their arrival in Switzerland.

6. **Which of the following statements is true about Norwegian Healthcare System?**

    a) National Health Service provides universal healthcare in Norway.

    b) About 10% of the Norwegian population is covered by private supplementary insurance.

    c) There are 1.8 specialists in hospitals or ambulatory care for every practicing primary care physician.

    d) There are few public hospitals in Norway.

7. **In Norway, under which scheme people register with one primary general practitioner?**

    a) Primary G.P. scheme

    b) Register G.P. scheme

    c) Regular G.P. scheme

    d) Connect with G.P. scheme

8. **Which of the following statements is false about Chinese Healthcare System?**

    a) Primary care is delivered mainly through village doctors and health workers in rural clinics.

    b) In China, coverage by publicly financed health insurance is near universal.

    c) Patients cannot see a specialist without a referral from a G.P.

    d) Mental care is provided by specialty psychiatric hospitals and clinics.

9. **Which of the following countries allows non licensed providers to care for the residents of rural areas?**

    a) United States

    b) Switzerland

    c) Germany

    d) China

10. Which of the following statements is false about Australian Healthcare System?

    a) Private Health Insurance offers more choice of providers and faster access to non- emergency services.

    b) Medicare Benefits Scheme includes hospital care, medical services etc.

    c) Pharmaceutical Benefits Scheme (MBS) provides pharmaceutical subsidies.

    d) Patients are able to choose their own specialist and are not required to be referred by their G.P. to receive MBS subsidies.

11. Which of the following provides universal coverage to all the residents of France?

    a) Statutory Health Insurance

    b) Mandatory Health Insurance

    c) Medicare

    d) Private Health Insurance

12. What is the ratio of G.P.s to specialists in New Zealand?

    a) 1:3

    b) 2:3

    c) 3:4

    d) None of the above

13. The Constitution of India makes which of the following responsible for provision of healthcare?

    a) Central Government

    b) Private Sector

    c) State Governments

    d) Citizens

14. In rural India, primary healthcare services are provided through a network of which of the following?

    a) Sub-Divisional Hospitals, District Hospitals and Mobile Medical Units.

    b) Medical Colleges and Medical Research Institutes.

    c) Nursing Homes and Multispecialty Clinics.

    d) Sub Centers, Primary Health Centers and Community Health Centers.

15. Which of the following countries has the highest healthcare spending as a percentage of GDP?

    a) Canada

    b) Sweden

    c) United States

    d) France

16. Which of the following countries has the highest breast cancer five year net survival rate (90%)?

    a) United States

    b) United Kingdom

    c) Netherlands

    d) New Zealand

17. Which of the following healthcare systems is known for utilization of healthcare resources?

    a) United States

    b) German

    c) Indian

    d) New Zealand

18. **Which of the following country's Regular GP Scheme has drastically improved patient-doctor stability as well as better GP accessibility?**

    a) China

    b) India

    c) Norway

    d) None of the above

19. **Among the following countries, which one has the lowest healthcare spending as a percentage of GDP?**

    a) Switzerland

    b) France

    c) Sweden

    d) India

20. **What are the types of health literacy?**

    a) Letters, words and numbers

    b) Oral, spoken and linguistic

    c) Print, oral and numerical

    d) Quantitative, written and spoken

21. **Which of the following is the ability to read and understand text, to locate and interpret information in documents, pictures, sign boards etc?**

    a) Read literacy

    b) Print literacy

    c) Linguistic literacy

    d) Text literacy

22. Which of the following helps in reading food and beverage labels, measuring blood glucose levels and measuring blood pressure?

a) Numerical literacy

b) Print literacy

c) Quantitative literacy

d) Numbers literacy

23. Which of the following is the ability to speak and to listen to health information?

a) Spoken literacy

b) Oral literacy

c) Linguistic literacy

d) None of the above

Answer key

1. (d)	2. (a)	3. (b)	4. (a)	5. (b)	6. (b)	7. (c)	8. (c)
9. (d)	10. (d)	11. (a)	12. (b)	13. (c)	14. (d)	15. (c)	16. (a)
17. (b)	18. (c)	19. (d)	20. (c)	21. (b)	22. (a)	23. (b)	

Chapter 2

Strategic Perspectives of Healthcare Leadership

Abstract

Healthcare leaders play an important role in formulating the strategy of an organization. This chapter discusses three strategic frameworks that can characterize Indian healthcare market. These strategic frameworks are used to understand the working of Indian hospital sector, pharmaceutical sector and medical device and diagnostics sector.

Introduction

WHO defines health as 'the state of complete physical, mental and social wellbeing and not merely the absence of disease and infirmity'.

To achieve this vision of health, healthcare leaders around the globe develop healthcare models, formulate policies and take initiatives that suit their country's requirements and culture.

Healthcare leaders have a primary responsibility to lead change and drive innovation. While designing innovative solutions, they have to face a lot of challenges like safety issues, health disparities, poor patient outcomes, lack of implementation of evidence based care etc.

Healthcare Strategic Planning

Healthcare strategic planning practices provide focus and direction to the healthcare organizations.

Following are the steps in healthcare strategic planning-

1. Establish a unique, far reaching vision

The vision should represent a long term commitment and should have a truly transformational effect on the organization.

2. Attack critical issues

Prioritize the most important issues and direct organizational energy and resources to address them.

3. Develop focused, clear strategies

Strategy development involves finding means that address critical issues and recognizing likely barriers and constraints. These means should lead to tangible end. The ends must be definable targets at a point in the future so that it is possible to measure progress, make adjustments along the way and facilitate accountability.

4. Differentiate from competition

It is important to be significantly different from the competitors in a way that consumers truly value.

5. Achieve real benefits

Strategic plans should target benefits realization from the outset and drive towards achieving more benefits throughout the process and into implementation.

Healthcare leaders must develop strategic plans that are dynamic in nature. The plan's strategies must be adjusted according to the needs of an organization.

Innovation and creativity manifest themselves in a number of ways in strategic planning. Healthcare leaders should seek inputs from all parts of the organization. A climate of receptivity for new ideas should be encouraged. Emphasis should be laid on looking at alternatives and generating options that are novel. High priority must be given to developing ideas that create new market space.

Strategic planning in healthcare must be a bottom up process rather than top down. The bottom up approach has many benefits like it allows more broad, substantial and meaningful participation in the planning process that leads to creativity and innovation.

Healthcare organizations with flexible, continuously improving planning processes are able to adapt more readily to the changing environment. Such organizations use external factors and create the platform for change which is necessary to keep strategic planning alive.

According to Richard Rumelt, strategy is about diagnosing a particular problem, finding a guiding policy and designing a set of coherent actions.

'Diagnosis' defines the nature of challenge. A good diagnosis identifies certain aspects of the situation that are critical. 'Guiding policy' is a general approach to overcome the obstacles identified in the diagnosis. 'Coherent actions' are the steps that coordinate with each other to work together in compliance with the guide.

Strategic Frameworks

Following are the three strategic frameworks that can help to characterize Indian healthcare market-

The first strategic framework is Porter's Five Forces which operate at the industry level. This framework helps to understand the level of competition within a given industry and the overall profitability of that industry.

According to Michael Porter, the nature of competition in any industry is determined by five forces-

- Existing competitors
- Potential entrants
- Substitutes
- Suppliers
- Buyers

1. Existing Competitors

Rivalry among existing competitors is intense when competitors are numerous and fairly equivalent in terms of size and power, when exit barriers are high and when industry growth is slow, resulting in struggle for market share. These characteristics are frequently observed in the healthcare market place, leading to intense rivalry within the industry.

2. Potential Entrants

Entities that might potentially enter the market represent a notable threat to existing competitors. New entrants bring new capacity and resources to the market along with a desire for market share. The magnitude of threat posed by new entrants largely depends on the particular barriers to entry that exist. Entry barriers provide protection from new entrants, while a few barriers increase competition in the market. Certificates of need possessed by hospitals and patent rights possessed by pharmaceutical firms are examples of barriers that offer substantial protection in the healthcare market place.

3. Substitutes

Substitutes are the products that differ from particular offerings but largely and sometimes completely fulfil equivalent wants and needs. As a result, substitute offerings can greatly impact the performance of healthcare entities and even threaten their very existence. The seriousness of threat of substitutes depends on their performance and price characteristics. Substitutes that offer equal or better performance give rise to considerable trouble especially when price advantages exist. Laser vision correction could be viewed as a substitute for eye glasses and contact lenses.

4. Suppliers

Suppliers provide the components necessary for healthcare organizations to offer goods and services to their customers. Surgery scalpels, pharmaceuticals, hospital beds and diagnostic imagery equipments represent just a few of the many products that healthcare entities purchase from suppliers. Without these 'raw materials', healthcare entities could not function. This dependence on suppliers causes serious risk to healthcare entities. Suppliers can raise the prices, lower the quality of components they provide or simply go out of business. All these situations can lead to potentially devastating effects. Suppliers are particularly powerful if they are few in number, if few substitutes exist, and if entities are not key customers.

5. Buyers

Porter's term 'buyers' is equivalent to the term customers, which is better suited for the healthcare market place. Customers possess significant bargaining power over healthcare entities because their patronage ultimately determines institutional survival, growth and prosperity. The array of customers in the healthcare market place is quite varied including residents in nursing homes, patients in hospitals, recipients of home healthcare services and even health insurance companies and other third party payer entities that pay for medical services on behalf of clients. Marketers must ensure that all marketing efforts are customer focussed. They must strive to assess accurately the wants and needs of customers and serve them in a manner that will meet and exceed their expectations.

The second strategic framework is the resource based view which operates at the firm level. This framework helps to analyze the competitive advantage of a specific firm within an industry.

In a resource based view model, resources are given the major role in helping companies to achieve higher organizational performance. There are two types of resources.

1. Tangible resources

Tangible resources are physical assets. They can be bought easily in the market so they confer little advantage to the companies in the long run because rivals can soon acquire the identical assets.

2. Intangible resources

Intangible resources are those that have no physical presence e.g. brand reputation, trademarks, intellectual property etc. These resources stay within a company and are the main source of sustainable competitive advantage.

The assumptions of resource based view are that the resources must also be heterogeneous and immobile.

The first assumption is that skills, capabilities and other resources that organizations possess differ from one company to another. If organizations would have the same amount and mix of resources, they could not employ different strategies to out compete each other. Therefore resource based view assumes that companies achieve competitive advantage by using their different bundles of resources.

The second assumption is that resources are not mobile and do not move from one company to another at least in short run. Due to this immobility, companies cannot replicate rival's resources and implement same strategies. Intangible resources such as brand equity, processes, knowledge or intellectual property are usually immobile.

Although, heterogeneous and immobile resources are critical in achieving competitive advantage, they are not enough alone if the firms want to sustain it. The VRIO test examines if resources are valuable, rare, costly to imitate and non-substitutable. The resources and capabilities that answer yes to all the questions are the sustained competitive advantages.

The third strategic framework is the institution based view which operates at the institution level. This framework helps to understand the impact of institutions and regulations on firms and industries.

Institution based view focuses on the dynamic interaction between institutions and organizations and considers strategic choices as the outcome of such an interaction. It implies that strategic choices are not only driven by industry conditions and firm capabilities but are also a reflection of the formal and informal constraints of a particular institutional framework that managers confront.

Indian Hospital Sector

In India, earlier the secondary and tertiary care was mainly provided by missionary hospitals and public sector. But in recent times, over the last 20 years, there is an entry by a lot of private corporate chains. The focus of these private hospitals is on product strategy. Some of them focus on eye care, some on cancer care, others on paediatric care and so on. Also there is some kind of vertical integration which is happening in this sector. e.g. HCG which is a cancer hospital is also getting into the production of cancer medicines. Similarly, some of the pharmaceutical companies are getting into the hospital space.

The nature of competition in the Indian hospital sector is oligopolistic where there are a few big players who are locally or geographically focussed and other smaller players like nursing homes. Healthcare services provided by large hospitals usually cost more due to the fact that larger, professionally managed hospitals provide high quality care and are compliant with existing regulations. On the other hand, small nursing homes and clinics can easily offer cheaper services because they have no regulatory pressure to be complaint with existing quality standards.

The hospital sector of India seems to be attractive and there are many unmet needs of patients that are required to be fulfilled. So, there is always a threat of new entrants and of substitutes.

Indian hospitals have a decent amount of bargaining power because they can choose from a number of suppliers including those from global market.

Patients have less bargaining power in the Indian hospital sector.

One of the key resources that Indian hospitals are lacking is physicians. Here qualified physicians are valuable, rare, inimitable resources and are without substitutes. Those Indian hospitals that manage to employ highly skilled and qualified physicians have sustained competitive advantage.

Institutions also play an important role in the context of Indian hospitals.

In recent times, one can witness two developments in the Indian hospital sector. The first is that the organizations which have developed low cost, high quality frugal innovation business models are expanding their operations in the international markets. It indicates that the organizations are maturing and there is a global acceptability of their models.

Following are some of the challenges healthcare organizations can expect to face if they decide to expand in international markets-

1. Maintaining the affordability of services.

2. The risk of dealing with a new regulatory mechanism.

3. Availability of physicians and nurses.

The second development is that the healthcare organizations are now launching their initial public offerings (IPOs). An organization would go IPO because it wants to raise money from a broader set of investors. Once the firm goes public, it has to operate with the interests of the shareholders in mind, helping to create a more formal corporate governance structure.

Indian Pharmaceutical Sector

India has emerged as a market leader in generic drugs. The Indian pharmaceutical industry has evoked very empathetic reactions from all around the world for over more than two decades for supplying generic medicines globally and thereby helping nations to reduce the cost of medicines. The most effective strategy to incentivize innovation within the pharmaceutical industry is to create environment with strong protection for intellectual property.

The Indian pharmaceutical industry has been strongly supported by the government of India. India signed the Trade Related Intellectual Property Agreement in 1995 saying that the country will implement a strong product patent recognizing regime from 2005.

From 1970 to 2005, there was a regime in the country that only recognized process patents, gave shorter patent life term which engendered the formation of reverse engineering skills.

After signing the TRIPS agreement in 2005, India has become product patent compliant like all other developed economies but there is a particular provision that continues to raise debates.

This particular provision is Section 3(d). Section 3(d) prohibits ever greening of drug patents and allows patents on variants of only those chemical compounds that show significant enhancement in therapeutic efficacy. Section 3(d) does not provide patent protection for incremental innovation. Section 3(d) can be used as an effective tool in restraining incremental inventions and prevent ever greening of patents. Ever greening of patents results in high drug prices which majority of the Indian population can't afford.

The 'leader' firms in the Indian pharmaceutical sector are those which trained their employees in such a way that they often use their knowledge to set up their own firms, driving a cycle of entrepreneurship and cluster formation.

Apart from innovation, intellectual property and entrepreneurship, the pharmaceutical industry also faces the key challenge of quality.

The global biopharmaceutical industry over the last 10 to 15 years has moved very dramatically towards launching and adopting biological drugs. In the context of India, there has not been much movement in this direction. Indian biopharmaceutical firms have been traditionally focusing on the chemistry capabilities and they are involved in reverse engineering and the production of chemistry based small molecule drugs. But there are few firms like Biocon and Intas Pharmaceuticals that are coming up with the capabilities to replicate versions of large molecule drugs known as biosimilars.

Three aspects determine the success of firms in the context of large molecule biotechnology driven drugs.

The first one is the science and innovation capabilities. Clinical trials are needed to establish the efficacy of these drugs. It requires investment.

The second aspect is the complementary capabilities. In the context of Indian pharmaceutical sector, complementary capabilities refer to well-trained sales and distribution force. They need to interact with the physicians and convince them that a particular drug is going to be more efficacious than the current small molecular chemistry driven drugs.

The third aspect is the vaccine production capabilities of the Indian pharmaceutical sector.

The Indian pharmaceutical sector has been slow to embrace the production of biologics and biosimilars because of the following reasons-

1. The development and production of these drugs require a high level of scientific expertise.

2. Unlike generic small molecule drugs, biologics and biosimilars must be validated through clinical trials, requiring a significant financial investment on the part of the manufacturer.

It can be concluded that the Indian pharmaceutical sector has developed strong reverse engineering skills because of the following reasons-

1. For over two decades, the intellectual property regime in the country recognized only process patents and not product patents.

2. India has a large pool of well trained chemists who can apply their skills towards understanding the molecular chemistry of drugs.

3. India has a low level of biological expertise required to develop new drug molecules.

Indian Medical Device and Diagnostics Sector

The nature of competition in the Indian medical device and diagnostics sector is oligopolistic. Multi National Companies like Philips, Siemens, GE, Cerner etc are the dominant players in this sector. They are competing with each other in different segments. There are also players from the domestic market who offer their alternatives as lower price disruptive products. The threat of substitutes and of new entrants is medium to high. The small component manufacturers who are supplying to the dominant multi-national players are not so powerful in terms of their bargaining abilities. The bargaining power of suppliers is low because most of the multi-national players in this sector are vertically integrated. The bargaining power of customers is also low in this sector, e.g. if a patient is subject to MRI scan, he/she has to go through it, there is no other alternative.

From the resource point of view, skilled manpower can give competitive advantage to the firms in medical device and diagnostics sector. It is crucial to retain manpower and avoid knowledge spill over. Quality is an important parameter in resource based view. Companies that choose to focus on quality may have products that are priced higher than their less quality conscious counterparts. It is important for companies to balance the requirements of affordability and access.

From the institution point of view, following are the regulatory challenges that a disruptive start-up in India's medical device and diagnostics sector can expect to face-

1. Lack of comprehensive set of regulations that apply to this sector.

2. Regulatory ignorance i.e. the regulator does not have sufficient knowledge to evaluate the merits of the product under review.

3. Conflicts of interest within regulators and medical boards that might influence the evaluation of a product.

In India, doctors prefer imported devices over domestically produced ones as the later are not certified by the government. Following would be the unintended consequences of this lack of certification-

1. There would be a great demand for second hand devices of foreign origin as compared to brand new locally produced devices.

2. There would be a greater incentive for the dumping of low quality foreign made products in the Indian market.

There are three aspects that need to be emphasized in the context of medical device and diagnostics sector of India.

The first one is that this market is fragmented in nature. There are around forty thousand to one hundred thousand pathology diagnostic labs in the country. But just about hundred to two hundred of them are certified by the National Certification Agency or by the College of American Pathologists. Indian medical device and diagnostics sector needs regulation.

The second aspect relates to intellectual property. It is important for firms in the medical device and diagnostics sector to have strong patents for their products because patents grant greater credibility to Indian firms which are looking to take their products to the global market place. Patents do not automatically grant companies the right to charge arbitrarily high prices, rather they grant a transient competitive advantage which is only valid till the term of the patent. The global market is more likely to adopt products that have strong intellectual property protection as this is also an assurance of the quality of science and research underlying the product.

The third aspect is competition in global market.

The potential disadvantages for start-ups from Indian medical device and diagnostics sector looking to enter the global market are-

1. Only a few of them have strong intellectual property arrangements.

2. The science underlying their innovative technologies tends to be fragile.

3. The global market in the medical device and diagnostics sector does not generally hold a favourable opinion of products emerging from India.

Importance of Regulation in Healthcare Industry

In healthcare industry, a regulator steps in because organizations are profit oriented; their aim is to maximize their profits. At the other end, patients are concerned about their own welfare. So, it is important to monitor the working of the organizations. Regulations are necessary to ensure that health services are provided as and where needed, without any bias. Regulation has a significant impact on a firm's competitive advantage.

In the context of Indian healthcare industry, regulation has three dimensions.

1. Firms can self-regulate themselves.

2. Firms can co-regulate themselves through their industry associations.

3. Firms can regulate by a policy maker.

Disruptive Innovation in Healthcare

The period in which incumbent firms do not innovate beyond the prevailing dominant design, represents a point in industry evolution where there can be potential entry of disruptive firms.

Disruption is good for Indian healthcare markets because of the following reasons-

1. It offers consumers more choices (potentially using technology) at better price points.

2. Producers (hospitals, pharmaceutical companies, medical device makers, insurers) make profit from disruption.

3. Supply can never meet demand which is growing at an exponential rate. Therefore disruptive thinking is necessary to propel non-linear growth.

Conclusion

India's hospital sector has seen a considerable change over the past few decades. Several private organizations have entered in this sector, bringing with them new business models that deliver high quality of service. Some of the private hospital chains are also looking to take their innovative business models in the international market.

In India, it is important for the private players to expand their footprint in rural areas also where most of the Indian population resides. In such areas they should strive to provide affordable quality care.

The Indian pharmaceutical sector has acquired the reputation of being the 'pharmacy of the world' because of its strength in producing low cost, high quality generic drugs. In this sector, there is a general movement away from small molecule chemistry based drugs to larger biologics and biosimilars.

For this sector, the government should provide financial assistance so that pharmaceutical firms can establish labs where clinical trials may be done.

The Indian medical device and diagnostics market lacks strong intellectual property arrangements.

In this sector, there is a need of creating and protecting intellectual property. The government should promote regulation and create norms and standards.

References

1. Mumford, M.D., Scott, G.M., Gaddis, B. & Strange, J.M. (2002). Leading Creative People: Orchestrating Expertise and Relationships. *The Leadership Quarterly, 13,* 705-730.

2. Amabile, T.M., Mukti, K. (Oct, 2008). Creativity and the Role of Leader. *Harvard Business Review,* 1-13.

3. Fairholm, M.R. (2009). Leadership and Organizational Strategy. *The Innovation Journal: The Public Sector Innovation Journal, 14(1),* 1-13.

4. Porter, M. (Jan, 2008). The Five Competitive Forces that shape Strategy. *Harvard Business Review.*

5. Burns, L.R. (2014). *India's Healthcare Industry: Innovation in Delivery, Financing and Manufacturing.* Cambridge University Press.

6. Rezaie et al. (2012). Emergence of Biopharmaceuticals Innovators in China, India, Brazil and South Africa as global competitors and collaborators. Health *Research Policy and Systems,* 10-18.

7. Saberwal, & Gayatri. (Jan 25, 2016). India's Intellectual Property Based Biomedical Startups. *Current Science,* 110-20.

8. Chesbrough, H. (April-June, 2010). Business Model Innovation: Opportunities and Barriers. *Long Range Planning, 43(2-3),* 354-63.

9. Al-Sawai, A. (2013). Leadership of Healthcare Professionals: Where do we stand?. *Oman Med. J, 28,* 285-87.

10. Vance, C., & Larson, E. (2002). Leadership Research in Business and Healthcare. *J. Nurs. Scholarsh, 34,* 165-71.

11. Reich, M.R., Javadi, D., & Ghaffar, A. (2016). Introduction to the Special Issue on Effective Leadership for Health Systems. *Health System Reform, 2(3),* 171-75.

MCQs

1. **Which of the following is the correct definition of 'health' given by WHO?**

   a) Absence of disease

   b) Physical, mental and social well being

   c) The state of complete physical, mental and social well being and not merely the absence of disease and infirmity.

   d) Well being of mind, body and soul

2. **Which of the following statements is false about healthcare strategic planning?**

   a) The vision should represent a short term commitment.

   b) Give priority to most important issues.

   c) Develop focused and clear strategies.

   d) Develop dynamic strategic plans.

3. **Which of the following is the definition of 'strategy' given by Richard Rumelt?**

   a) Creating a long term vision statement for your organization.

   b) Diagnosing a particular problem, finding a guiding policy and designing a set of coherent actions.

   c) Analyzing your competitor's business model to identify strengths and weaknesses.

   d) Short term plan

4. **Which of the following is not the part of Porter's Five Forces framework?**

   a) Existing competitors

   b) Potential entrants

   c) Substitutes

   d) Technology used by competitors.

5. Which of the following is a tangible resource?

a) Trademarks

b) Intellectual property

c) Brand reputation

d) Well equipped building

6. What is the function of a VRIO test?

a) To examine if resources are versatile, reliable, costly to imitate and non- substitutable.

b) To examine if resources are valuable, rare, imitable and substitutable.

c) To examine if resources are valuable, rare, costly to imitate and non- substitutable.

d) None of the above

7. According to the institution based view, which of the following is a vulnerability that firms must be prepared to address?

a) Dependence on specialized technology.

b) Changes in government policy that affect the way firms do business.

c) Cheaper products developed by competitors.

d) Inefficient bundling of resources that reduces core competence.

8. Which of the following statements is true about Indian hospital sector?

a) Focus of the Indian private hospitals is on process strategy.

b) Nature of competition in this sector is monopolistic.

c) There is some kind of horizontal integration which is happening in this sector.

d) None of the above

9. **Which of the following statements is false about Indian hospital sector?**

   a) In this sector, there is always a threat of new entrants and of substitutes.

   b) Indian hospitals have a decent amount of bargaining power.

   c) Patients have less bargaining power in this sector.

   d) None of the above

10. **Why is there a global acceptability of Indian hospital models?**

   a) They are often headed by medical entrepreneurs.

   b) They can handle large amount of patients.

   c) They offer new business models capable of providing high quality care while keeping costs low.

   d) None of the above

11. **What are the reasons an Indian healthcare organization might choose to launch its Initial Public Offering?**

   a) It wants to raise money from a broader set of investors.

   b) Once the firm goes public, it has to operate with the interests of the share holders in mind, helping to create a more formal corporate governance structure.

   c) Both (a) and (b)

   d) None of the above

12. **India has emerged as a market leader in which of the following?**

   a) Brand name drugs

   b) Generic drugs

   c) Ayurvedic drugs

   d) None of the above

13. **What is the most effective strategy to incentivize innovation within the pharmaceutical industry?**

    a) Create an environment with strong protection for intellectual property.

    b) Offer prizes to companies that come up with new drugs.

    c) Prevent large global pharmaceutical players from selling their products in the Indian market.

    d) Prevent generic drug manufacturers from selling lower priced versions of drugs.

14. **In the context of intellectual property, which of the following statements is false about Section 3(d)?**

    a) It prohibits ever greening of drug patents.

    b) It allows patents on variants of only those chemical compounds that show significant enhancement in therapeutic efficacy.

    c) It provides patent protection for incremental innovation.

    d) None of the above

15. **Which of the following is not the aspect that determines the success of firms in the context of large molecule biotechnology driven drugs?**

    a) Science and innovation capabilities

    b) Chemistry capabilities

    c) Complementary capabilities

    d) Vaccine production capabilities

16. **The Indian pharmaceutical sector has been slow to embrace the production of biologics and biosimilars because of which of the following reasons?**

    a) Their production requires a high level of scientific expertise.

    b) Biologics and biosimilars must be validated through clinical trials.

    c) Significant financial investment is required on the part of the manufacturer.

    d) All of the above

17. **Which of the following is not the reason for the development of strong reverse engineering skills in the context of Indian pharmaceutical sector?**

    a) From 1970-2005, there was a regime in the country that only recognized product patents.
    b) India has a large pool of well trained chemists.
    c) India has a low level of biological expertise required to develop new drug molecules.
    d) None of the above

18. **In the context of the Indian pharmaceutical sector, complementary capabilities refer to:**

    a) A well trained sales and distribution force
    b) Research and development capabilities
    c) Entry by new entrepreneurs
    d) Tie-ups with physicians to market products

19. **Why do big multi-national players in the Indian medical device and diagnostics sector have a higher bargaining power with the suppliers?**

    a) They have a greater competitive advantage compared to smaller firms in this sector.
    b) They tend to be vertically integrated.
    c) They have access to suppliers in multiple markets around the world.
    d) They have greater financial resources that enable them to be more competitive.

20. **Which of the following statements is false about the Indian medical device and diagnostics sector?**

    a) In this sector, the nature of competition is oligopolistic.
    b) The threat of substitutes and of new entrants is medium to high.
    c) The bargaining power of suppliers is low.
    d) The bargaining power of customers is high.

21. Which of the following is a potential disadvantage for healthcare tech start-ups from India looking to enter the global market?

a) The global market in the medical device and diagnostics sector does not generally hold a favourable opinion of products emerging from India.

b) Only a few of such healthcare tech start-ups have strong intellectual property arrangements.

c) The science underlying their innovative technologies tends to be fragile.

d) All of the above.

22. Which of the following represents a point in industry evolution where there can be potential entry of disruptive firms?

a) The period in which a few incumbent firms within the industry establish the dominant design.

b) The period in which there is some turmoil within the industry and several firms exit.

c) The period in which incumbent firms do not innovate beyond the prevailing dominant design.

d) The period in which several firms enter the industry.

Answer key

1. (c) 2. (a) 3. (b) 4. (d) 5. (d) 6. (c) 7. (b) 8. (d)

9. (d) 10. (c) 11. (c) 12. (b) 13. (a) 14. (c) 15. (b) 16. (d)

17. (a) 18. (a) 19. (b) 20. (d) 21. (d) 22. (c)

Chapter 3

Quality and Safety Issues in Healthcare Facility

Abstract

The foremost aim of any healthcare organization should be to provide safe and quality care to the patients. This chapter discusses the causes of error in the hospital, the safety measures that can be taken to avoid them and the generic techniques to minimize hospital infection. The methods to measure quality and the ways to improve it have also been explored in this chapter.

Introduction

It is not easy to define quality and when one is asked to define 'healthcare quality', it becomes even more difficult. 'Perception' is involved in defining quality. A person perceives that quality is achieved only when he/she is fully satisfied. Quality is also dynamic in nature which requires improvements at regular intervals. So, quality means satisfying customer on a continuous basis.

Healthcare Quality

In order to achieve healthcare quality, it is important to consider the satisfaction level of all the stakeholders involved like patients, clinicians, health insurance companies etc.

Patient and clinician satisfaction can be attained through expected 'health outcomes'. 'Standardization' of processes and procedures can lead to expected health outcomes.

According to Avedis Donabedian, healthcare quality can also be seen as a 'structure', 'process' and 'outcome'.

'Structure' is the context in which care is delivered. It includes physical facility, equipments and human resources, as well as organizational characteristics such as staff training and payment methods. These factors control how healthcare providers act in a healthcare system and are measures of the average quality of care within a facility.

It can pose the following questions-

1. Is hospital well equipped?

2. Are physicians qualified?

3. Are they accreditated and licensed?

4. Is the nursing staff trained?

'Process' refers to the way of giving care.

It includes diagnosis, treatment, preventive care and patient education.

It can pose the following questions-

1. Are physicians doing the right procedure?

2. Are nurses following the protocols?

3. Are they using the right preventive measures to avoid infections?

'Outcomes' are about the states of health that patients achieve. It includes changes to health status, behavior or knowledge as well as patient satisfaction and health related quality of life.

It can pose the following questions-

1. Did the patient develop an infection during his/her stay at the hospital?

2. Did the patient actually come out of the hospital with a good experience?

According to Institute of Medicine (IOM), healthcare quality has six aims-

1. Safety

Health care cannot be of high quality if it is unsafe. Safe care refers to delivering health care that avoids injury to patients. Safe care aims to reduce the risks involved in healthcare delivery process.

2. Effectiveness

It refers to providing care based on scientific knowledge. The healthcare organizations should prefer evidence based practices for improving health outcomes.

3. Efficiency

It refers to avoiding waste through judicious use of healthcare resources.

4. Timeliness

It implies reducing waiting time for recipients of care and delivering health care in a timely manner.

5. Patient centered

It means providing responsive care which ensures that patient values guide clinical decisions.

6. Equality

It implies ensuring that the quality of care does not vary from person to person on the grounds of gender, race, religion, ethnicity, socio-economic background or geographic location. Similar quality of healthcare should be provided to all.

ISO 9000 Series of Standards

ISO 9000: 1987

In 1987, the International Organization for Standardization (ISO) developed and published ISO 9000 series of International Standards on Quality Management System.

ISO 9000: 1994

The 1994 version laid emphasis on quality assurance through preventive actions and acquired evidence of compliance with documented procedures.

ISO 9000: 2000

The 2000 version introduced the concept of 'process management'. The quality management approach in these standards focuses on analyzing the customer's requirements and defining 'processes' that contribute to the achievement of a product which is acceptable to the customer.

ISO 9000: 2000 Series of Quality Standards comprises of the following three standards:

(i) ISO 9000: 2000 standard defines the 'fundamentals' and 'terminology' used in ISO 9000 series of standards.

(ii) ISO 9001:2000 defines the 'requirements' needed by an organization to demonstrate its ability to provide products and services that meet customer's demands and enhance their satisfaction.

(iii) ISO 9004:2000 provides 'guidelines' for improving the performance of an organization.

ISO 9000 series of standards is revised after every 4-6 years.

The principles and structure of ISO 9000 can be applied to healthcare also.

Compliance to ISO 9000 Series of Standards derives some of the following benefits for healthcare organizations-

1. ISO 9000 provides opportunities to standardize the service throughout the healthcare organization.

2. ISO 9000 has potential for efficiency gains and cost reduction because of its process orientation.

3. ISO 9000 advocates the importance of review and continual improvement.

4. ISO 9000 has the potential to make accreditation and conformity to other requirements much simpler.

Since ISO 9000 series of standards is 'process oriented', 'customer focused' and demands 'continual improvement', it ensures reliable and better quality of healthcare.

Accreditation

Accreditation in healthcare is important to set standards for delivering healthcare services. Accreditation doesn't restrict innovation and diversity in service delivery. It only helps in guiding the healthcare providers to maintain quality that leads to better results and outcomes.

Accreditation in healthcare system refers to the systematic assessment of hospitals against accepted standards.

Optimum standards, professional accountability and continual excellence are the basis for accreditation. Accreditation paves the way to develop hospital framework for establishing structure, identifying processes and measuring outcomes that ensure delivery of quality care. Once hospital is found to be complying with the accreditation standards, the national accreditation body grants certificate of accreditation.

Joint Commission International (JCI)

It works to improve patient safety and quality of healthcare in the international community by offering education, publications, advisory services and international accreditation and certification.

Following are the 10 stages that lead to JCI accreditation success-

1. Become familiar with JCI's accreditation standards and survey process.

2. Conduct gap analysis and build action plan.

3. Update policies and procedures.

4. Target improvements where needed.

5. Work with staff to overcome obstacles.

6. Assess your readiness at the midpoint.

7. Continue training for sustainable changes.

8. Evaluate and refine processes.

9. Use a mock survey to assess your readiness.

10. Make final modifications.

Following are some of the areas that are covered under the Joint Commission International accreditation process-

1. Two patient identifiers

2. Hand washing

3. Medication regulation

4. Fall precautions

5. Workspace area

6. Hospital airflow

7. Patient handoffs

8. Staffing ratios

National Accreditation Board for Hospitals and Healthcare Providers (NABH)

It is a constituent board of Quality Council of India. It is established to enhance the quality of healthcare system in India. NABH standards provide framework for quality assurance and quality improvement for public and private healthcare providers.

NABH standards are divided into the following 10 areas-

Patient Centered Standards

1. Access, Assessment and Continuity of Care (ACC)

2. Care of Patients (COP)

3. Management of Medication (MOM)

4. Patient Rights and Education (PRE)

5. Hospital Infection Control (HIC)

Organization Centered Standards

6. Continuous Quality Improvement (CQI)

7. Responsibility of Management (ROM)

8. Facility Management and Safety (FMS)

9. Human Resource Management (HRM)

10. Information Management System (IMS)

NABH accreditation helps healthcare planners to evaluate their healthcare systems and make desired changes accordingly.

Accreditation is voluntary while Regulation is mandatory. Regulation ensures minimum standards. In terms of quality, regulation denotes minimum quality while accreditation symbolizes optimum quality.

In hospitals, healthcare professionals, buildings, equipments all are subject to regulation.

Licensing is one set of regulatory mechanisms. The idea behind licensing is that if a doctor is going to practice medicine, he or she needs to have met minimum training requirements.

Healthcare professionals such as doctors, nurses, pharmacists etc. need central/state level registrations in order to provide services.

National Medical Commission Bill, 2019 introduces a common final year undergraduate examination called the National Exit Test for the students graduating from medical institutions to obtain the license for practice.

Both regulation and accreditation play important role in ensuring patient safety and quality of care.

Patient Safety

WHO defines patient safety as the 'absence of preventable harm to a patient during the process of health care and reduction of risk of unnecessary harm associated with health care to an acceptable minimum'.

Hospital systems are complex because of the involvement of several people, processes, equipments and their inter-dependencies. Slight negligence and unintentional human error can become fatal for the patients.

43 million people around the world are injured every year due to unsafe medical care that just happens in hospitals. According to a study, in India, 5.2 million medical errors are happening annually.

Causes of Error

Following are the main causes of error in the hospitals-

1. Hospital Acquired Infections (Nosocomial Infections)

It is an infection acquired in the hospital by a patient in whom the infection was not present or incubating at the time of admission.

At any given time, over 1.4 million people across the globe suffer a nosocomial infection.

Hospital acquired infections are far more common in India than in Western countries. This occurs at an alarming rate of one infection per four hospital visits compared to one in ten for European country and one in twenty for the United States.

In India, many factors contribute to nosocomial infections like use of unsafe injections, lack of cleanliness in hospital settings, poor quality of dietary services etc.

Hospital acquired infections may be caused by a micro-organism acquired from another person in the hospital (cross infection), or by patient's own endogenous flora (endogenous infection) or may be acquired from a substance recently contaminated from another human source (environmental infection).

A patient's susceptibility of acquiring infection depends on his/her age, immune system, underlying disease and diagnostic and therapeutic procedures.

Following are the common hospital acquired infections-

(a) Catheter Related Blood Stream Infections

Since catheters are inserted into the venous or arterial blood stream, they bypass normal skin defense mechanism and hence provide a path for micro-organisms to enter the blood stream.

Safety Measures

(i) Avoid catheterization unless there is a medical indication.

(ii) Limit the use of catheters to duration as short as possible.

(iii) Hands must be washed before all catheter care.

(iv) Prepare fluids aseptically and immediately before use. The infusion container should be inspected for faults, leaks, cloudiness or particulate matter before connected to the drip set and if any of these are present, it must be discarded.

(v) A high level of aseptic technique should be used for insertion and handling of catheters.

(vi) Skin at the insertion site should be thoroughly disinfected with an anti-septic solution.

(vii) Change dressing at the time of change of lines following surgical asepsis.

(b) Urinary Tract Infections

In hospitals, there is a high incidence of catheter related urinary tract infections. The main cause of these infections is the indwelling catheter which is inserted into the bladder and allowed to remain in it .e.g. Foley catheter

Safety Measures

(i) Urinary catheters should be inserted only when extremely needed. Prolonged catheterization should be avoided.

(ii) They should be inserted using aseptic technique and sterile equipment.

(iii) Anti-septic solution for periurethral cleaning and a single use packet of lubricant jelly should be used for insertion.

(iv) Small catheters should be used to minimize urethral trauma.

(v) Closed sterile drainage system should be maintained.

(c) Surgical Site Infections

It is an infection at the surgical site that occurs within 30 days of the surgical procedure or within one year if there is an implant.

Some of the infections at the site of an open incision are deep and some are superficial ones.

Safety Measures

(i) Pre-operative anti-septic bath

(ii) Pre-operative skin preparation

(iii) Maintain high level of asepsis during surgery.

(iv) Boost immunity if possible.

(v) Avoid long stay in hospitals.

(d) Clostridium Difficile Infections

These occur in the gut. These infections happen most often when the patient has been exposed to an antibiotic. Clostridium difficile infections can cause very serious diarrhea.

Chemotherapy drugs can cause clostridium difficile infections.

Safety Measures

(i) Avoid broad spectrum antibiotics.

(ii) Hospital kitchen hygiene should be maintained to provide good quality food to the patients.

(e) Nosocomial Pneumonia

The greatest incidence of purulent tracheobronchitis and pneumonia as nosocomial infections is in patients who have received ventilator assistance.

Safety Measures

(i)   Aseptic techniques should be used in handling endotracheal tubes and tracheostomy tubes.

(ii) Catheter should be used only once.

(iii) Nurses should use sterile gloves for suctioning.

2.   Adverse Drug Event (ADE)

It is harm to the patient that is caused by a medication.

Adverse drug event includes adverse drug reactions, medication errors, allergic reactions, overdoses etc.

Adverse drug reaction is an unwanted, undesirable effect of a medication that occurs during usual clinical use. Examples of adverse drug reactions include rashes, jaundice, anemia, a decrease in the white blood cell count, kidney damage , nerve injury that may impair vision or hearing etc.

Medication error is an error at any step along the pathway that begins when a clinician prescribes a medication and ends when the patient actually receives it.

It includes errors that occur in selection and procurement of medicines, their storage, ordering and transcribing, preparing and dispensing, medication administering and monitoring patients after giving the medicine.

About 50% of the errors actually happen at ordering of medicine stage, 10% at transcribing stage, 10% at dispensing stage and nearly 30% at administering stage.

Safety Measures

(i) Ordering errors can be minimized using Computerized Physician Order Entry (CPOE) system. It enables doctors to write the order on a computer. This order is written by checking details like patient's age, his/her level of kidney function, reaction of the ordered drug with other drugs the patient is already taking etc. After all these checks, the order is written and it goes electronically directly to the pharmacy.

(ii) Reference material about doses and interaction should be made available on a webpage of the hospital website.

(iii) Errors that occur in pharmacy can be reduced by bar coding medicines.

(iv) Drug administration errors can be minimized by feeding information in smart pumps regarding what medication is being administered.

3. Fall

Generally, people don't have serious injury from fall but sometimes they do, like fractures or having bleeding. Sometimes they suffer subdural hematoma.

Causes of Fall

(i) Anything that makes patients confused.

(ii) If patient is incontinent (i.e. not being under control).

(iii) If patient is demented (i.e. unable to think or act clearly because of extreme worry or anger etc.).

Safety Measure

(i) Try to profile patients according to their risk of fall. If somebody is at high risk, then take fall precautions for him/her to minimize the likelihood of fall.

4. Pressure Ulcers

Pressure ulcer or bed sore is a sore that the patient gets from lying in one place for too long.

Safety Measure

(i) Make sure to turn the patients who are likely to develop pressure sores.

5. Deep Venous Thrombosis

It means developing a blood clot. They typically occur in veins usually in the legs. Sometimes clots move up to the lungs and cause pulmonary emboli and trouble breathing and even death. People who are at bed rest can develop deep venous thrombosis. So, immobility is the main risk factor.

Safety Measures

(i) To avoid deep venous thrombosis, use mechanical devices that keep the blood flow by squeezing the leg on a periodic basis.

(ii) Anti-coagulants can be given to avoid deep venous thrombosis.

6. Surgical Complications

Surgical complications include wrong site or wrong patient surgery, retained foreign objects, or complications due to incorrect technique, failure of equipment or insufficient training of staff.

Safety Measures

(i) Only qualified and trained surgeons should be allowed to perform complicated surgeries.

(ii) Extreme care should be taken while performing operations.

(iii) Patients should not be discharged early after surgery because post-operative care is very important.

(iv) After discharge, physicians should persuade patients for follow ups.

Generic Techniques to Minimize Infection

Following are some of the generic techniques that can be followed to minimize infection in the hospitals-

1. Hand hygiene

2. Aseptic techniques

3. Standard precautions

4. Airborne precautions

5. Droplet precautions

6. Contact precautions

7. Disinfection techniques

8. Surveillance

1. Hand Hygiene

There are three levels of hand hygiene

(i) Routine hand wash

(ii) Anti-septic hand wash

(iii) Surgical scrub

(i) Routine Hand Wash

It involves applying soap thoroughly over the hands, rubbing fingers together back and forth for 15 to 30 seconds, rinsing hands under a stream of running water until all soap is gone and drying hands with a clean single use towel.

(ii) Antiseptic Hand Wash

It means washing hands with anti-septic preparations (iodophors or chlorhexidine) or with alcohol based anti-septic hand rubs.

Anti-septic hand wash reduces concentration of resident flora as well as inactivates transient micro-organisms from hands.

(iii) Surgical Scrub

It involves first decontaminating the hands then donning a sterile surgical gown and a pair of sterile gloves.

2. Aseptic Techniques

Aseptic techniques involve practices that minimize the introduction of microorganisms to patients during patient care.

There are two categories of asepsis

    (i) Medical Asepsis

    (ii) Surgical Asepsis

(i) Medical Asepsis

It is also known as clean technique. It is concerned with eliminating the spread of micro-organisms through facility practices.

(ii) Surgical Asepsis

It is also known as sterile technique. It is the absence of all microorganisms within any type of invasive procedure. It aims to maintain a sterile field for surgery.

According to Joint Commission International, there are four aspects of aseptic technique

    (a) Barriers- They protect the patient from the transfer of pathogens from a healthcare worker, from the environment or from both.

    Some of the barriers used in aseptic technique are sterile gloves, gowns and drapes, masks for patients and healthcare providers etc.

    (b) Patient Equipment and Preparation- Healthcare providers should use sterile equipments and instruments.

(c) Environmental Controls- Maintain a sterile environment around the patient.

(d) Contact guidelines- Once healthcare providers have put on sterile barriers, they should avoid touching non sterile items.

3. Standard Precautions

Following are the WHO healthcare facility recommendations for standard precautions-

(i) Hand hygiene

(ii) Gloves

(iii) Facial protection (eye, nose and mouth)

(iv) Gown

(v) Prevention of needle stick and injuries from other sharp instruments

(vi) Respiratory hygiene and cough etiquettes

(vii) Environmental cleaning

(viii) Linens

(ix) Waste disposal

(x) Patient care equipment

4. Airborne Precautions

Airborne transmission occurs when droplet nuclei <5 micron in size are disseminated in air. Diseases that spread by this mode include pulmonary TB, measles, chickenpox, pulmonary plague etc.

Following precautions should be taken while entering the air borne isolation room-

(i) Place the patient in a negative pressure room. Negative pressure allows air to flow into isolation room but not escape from it. It prevents contaminated air from escaping the room.

(ii) Anyone who enters isolation room must wear a special high filtration, particulate respirator (e.g. N95 mask).

(iii) Limit the movement and transport of patients from the room. They should be moved for essential purposes only.

5. Droplet Precautions

These are used for a patient who is infected with micro-organisms transmitted by large droplet (>5 micron in size) that can be generated by the patient during coughing, sneezing, talking or while performing procedures that involve respiratory tract. Micro-organisms can be acquired by direct contact, by contact with droplets over a distance up to 6 feet as well as by contact with objects recently contaminated with respiratory secretions.

Diseases which are transmitted by this route include pneumonias, pertussis, diphtheria, influenza, mumps, meningitis etc.

Following precautions should be taken-

(i) Place the patient in a single room or in a room with another patient infected by the same pathogen.

(ii) Wear a surgical mask when working within 1-2 meters of the patient (3-6 feet).

(iii) Wear a non-sterile gown when working within 3-6 meters of the patient.

(iv) Place a surgical mask on the patient if transport is necessary.

6. Contact Precautions

These are used for patients who are infected with organisms that can be transmitted by direct contact with the patient while performing patient care activities that require touching the patient's dry skin or indirect contact with environmental surfaces or patient care items.

Diseases that are transmitted by this route include colonization or infection with multiple antibiotic resistant organisms, enteric infections and skin infections.

Following precautions should be taken-

(i)   Place the patient in a single room or in a room with another patient infected by the same pathogen.

(ii) Wear clean, non sterile gloves when entering the room.

(iii) Wear a clean, non sterile gown when entering the room if substantial contact with the patient, environmental surfaces or items in the patient's room is anticipated.

(iv) Limit the movement and transport of patients from the room. They should be moved for essential purposes only.

(v)   Draining wounds should be covered with clean dressing.

7. Disinfection Techniques

(i)   For terminal disinfection of isolation rooms and operating rooms, fogging with incidur and hydrogen peroxide should be used.

(ii) The floors of rooms and washrooms should be cleaned with soap and water and a disinfectant should be used.

(iii) Portable water needs to be used for any kitchen activity. Reverse osmosis or treated water should be used for drinking. Cleaning of the water storage tank should be done on regular basis. Treated water should be used for cleaning of utensils and preparation of food.

8. Surveillance

Surveillance is important to ensure that an infection control program is functioning properly.

While developing a surveillance program, one should consider the characteristics of an institution, including size, hospital type, patient population served, procedures and treatment offered and proportion of inpatient to outpatient care. It is also important to consider the resources available to the infection control program, including budget, number of personnel, their level of training and experience.

Quality Measurement

It requires defining the 'quality' first. It means developing standards of quality. These standards are the expected levels of performance. After establishing standards, quality can be measured by comparing actual outcomes against the desired outcomes. Quality measurement serves as an input for quality improvement. Healthcare quality measurement quantifies healthcare processes, outcomes, organizational structures that are deployed to provide quality care.

Following are some of the metrics for measuring the quality of care in hospital settings:

1. Consultation Time

Consultation time can bridge the 'know do gap'.

In terms of healthcare, it is a gap between what the doctor can do and what he/she actually does in terms of treatment given to the patients.

The more time a physician spends with a patient, the more things he/she will do which he/she should do for that patient.

2. Number of questions the doctor asked about patient's health

If the doctor spends more time interacting with a patient, listen carefully to the medical history, then he/she will definitely give a better advice.

3. Number of physical exams that he or she did

Mobile technology can be used to get the above information from patients.

Indicators

In the Indian healthcare scenario, after the onset of national accreditation, there has been a huge movement towards setting up the structures and processes associated with quality.

Rather than health outcomes, the concept of indicators to monitor clinical and managerial efficiency and effectiveness has taken root in Indian healthcare system.

An indicator can be defined as a statistical measure of the performance of functions, systems or processes overtime.

Indicators are broadly classified into two categories

a) Clinical indicators

b) Managerial indicators

(a) Clinical Indicators

They are chosen from areas of patient assessment and care, laboratory and radiology safety parameters and test turn-around-time, anesthesia indicators, infection control parameters, medication management indicators including medication errors and stock outs, surgical outcomes, emergency response time etc.

(b) Managerial Indicators

These are chosen from patient satisfaction indices, employee satisfaction indices, length of stay, equipment downtime, critical area utilization etc.

Various indicators are defined in the chapter on Quality Improvement and Patient Safety of the 4th edition of Joint Commission International (JCI) standards and in the chapter on Continuous Quality Improvement of the 3rd edition of National Accreditation Board for Hospitals and Healthcare Providers (NABH) standards.

All indicators must be viewed as a trend over time. This helps the quality practitioners to determine whether any deviation from the trend is a common cause variation or a special cause variation because treatment to both of them is different.

Defining appropriate indicators, collecting and collating data, representing them as trends over time and implementing quality improvement initiatives represents the complete cycle of quality management.

Following indicators can be used in health care systems-

For Primary Care (Ambulatory Care)	(i) Admission rate for chronic diseases e.g. look at how good is the system in avoiding the people with COPD, asthma, diabetes, chronic heart failure in a hospital.
	(ii) Prescription indicators e.g. look at antibiotic prescribing. Look at the third and fourth generation antibiotics as a percentage of the whole.
For Acute Care	(i) 40 day case fatality rates for stroke
For Breast Cancer, Cervical Cancer, Colon Cancer	(i) Five year survival rate (ii) Mortality rate (iii) Screening rate
For Mental Health care	(i) Look at the life expectancy rate of people who were once been diagnosed with schizophrenia or bipolar disorder.

Quality measurement is dependent on the capability of an organization to link different databases and its ability to maximize the use of data captured in electronic health records. So, for quality measurement, it is important to strengthen the information infrastructure to capture the data.

How the healthcare organization is performing in terms of quality can be measured if it maintains data at each level of care delivery.

The countries that lack pre-existing data infrastructure can measure quality through the patient's feedback. So, such countries need to focus on 'patient experience management' and strive to increase patient satisfaction. Real-time patient feedback can be used to assess the patient's level of satisfaction. Plan-Do-Study-Act (PDSA) cycle can be implemented in getting patient feedback.

Plan: Distribute feedback forms among patients waiting for their turn in OPD.

Do: Coordinate the process of filling the forms.

Study: Analyze the results of survey and find out the areas which need improvement.

Act: Implement desired changes in the system in order to provide better services to the patients.

Quality Improvement

In order to improve quality three things are needed

a) Will

b) New ideas

c) Execution skills

Quality in the healthcare sector can be improved if an organization has a will to make it perform best.

For improving performance, the organization must come up with new ideas and employ its workforce to execute them in an effective manner.

The role of leadership in healthcare quality improvement is to see what the care is, what the care should be and to improve accordingly.

Following are some of the ways through which healthcare quality can be improved-

1. Balancing under treatment and overtreatment

From the Indian healthcare perspective, in public sector, there is an acute shortage of healthcare providers and infrastructure which leads to under treatment of patients. So, in public sector, linking treatment with payment can improve the quality of treatment given to patients. In private sector, doctors may prescribe costly surgical procedures and medicines which are otherwise not needed. Some laboratories offer kickbacks to doctors who refer patients to their diagnostic centers. So, in private sector, it is not a good idea to link treatment with payment.

2. Follow up

It is an important part of treatment because its negligence can cause greater harm in the long run. Generally physicians ask patients to follow strictly the prescribed medication and encourage them for follow ups.

Healthcare organizations should create a system that can remind patients about follow ups through sending a message on their registered mobile numbers.

3. Only qualified and trained doctors should be allowed to become practitioners. There should be no corruption in issuing practicing license to the doctors. Patients should avoid visiting those practitioners who don't have practicing license.

4. Doctors should devote more time per patient in order to make a right diagnosis.

5. The diagnostic tools used by doctors should be in good state.

6. Protocolization

The more protocolization we bring in the healthcare system, the more we can do, the better the care is going to become.

7. Accountability

If a doctor is made accountable for what he/she does in terms of treatment, better results can be expected.

Strategic Quality Planning

Strategic planning is the process of laying down long and short term organizational objectives based on the organization's mission and vision, identifying and providing ways and means to achieve them and measuring the effectiveness of such efforts for continual improvement. It is the responsibility of the leaders of an organization to do strategic planning.

Healthcare leaders do strategic quality planning to render quality healthcare services.

Following leadership groups can be found in healthcare industries-

(i) Governing Body/Council

(ii) Chief Executive Officer

(iii) Quality Head/ Coordinator

(iv) Chief Nursing Superintendent

(v) Heads of various clinical and diagnostic service departments

(vi) Heads of other support service departments

Collaborative style of leadership is effective in strategic quality planning in healthcare organizations.

Following are the three responsibilities of leadership in strategic quality planning-

1. Strategy Formulation

Strategy is formulated on the basis of mission, vision and value statements of an organization. Mission statement describes the purpose of existence of an organization. Vision statement declares where an organization wants to be. Value statement depicts the principles of an organization. Strategy formulation starts with identifying the stakeholder's requirements and expectations and seeking their involvement in the quality implementation plan.

External environment analysis is done to find out the available opportunities and challenges prevailing in the market.

Internal environment analysis is done to figure out the strengths and weaknesses of an organization.

Gap analysis is done to identify the gaps between the current state and the future state of an organization. The next step is to involve all stake holders for developing a plan to close the gaps. The plan should be aligned with the mission, vision and core values of an organization.

2. Strategy Implementation

It is the stage of executing the plan. It involves resource allocation, designing change, overcoming resistance to change, communicating and collaborating with all the people concerned. So, at this stage, a leader has to play the role of a facilitator and communicator as well as a change agent and negotiator.

3. Strategy Monitoring and Evaluation

This stage involves monitoring activity and assessing progress. It is the responsibility of the leadership to review the progress of implementation stage based on the pre-determined timeliness, modifying it whenever needed and communicating the progress to the interested parties.

Team Building

One of the most significant roles of leadership in framing the strategy for quality improvement is building teams. Quality improvement cannot be achieved by one person working alone or groups of persons working in an uncoordinated manner. There is a requirement of having a team that maintains, sustains and coordinates the quality movement. It is the responsibility of the leadership to choose a team that implements quality driven strategy.

In healthcare organizations, there are many activities that need to take place and several specific areas of expertise have to be covered. So, it is essential to set 'sub teams'. The various quality teams in a healthcare organization are quality improvement teams, patient safety teams, infection control teams, clinical audit teams etc.

Communication

Effective communication is important to support all the facets of strategic quality planning. Communication helps leadership to involve people, introduce innovations and quality improvement programs, introduce policies, procedures and protocols and get timely feedback.

Healthcare leaders should create an environment that encourages accountability and commitment. They should strive to develop a 'quality culture' in the healthcare organization by making it more 'patient centric'.

Conclusion

In India, both public and private sectors play an important role in providing and improving healthcare facilities and services.

Government opens medical colleges and hospitals, organizes immunization programs, encourages integration of IT in healthcare, provides financial assistance to healthcare institutions, arranges free health checkups, certifies practitioners, allocates health budgets for states etc. Private sector contributes to healthcare by establishing world class super specialty hospitals that provide quality care to the patients.

In India, healthcare reforms can be done in many areas like accessibility, affordability and quality of healthcare, doctor patient ratio, accountability of doctors, health insurance policies etc.

For poor sections of the society, healthcare should be less costly and more accessible.

Government should open more medical colleges to improve doctor patient ratio.

Laws should be made that can hold doctors accountable for medical errors.

Public private partnership is required for providing insurance plans to the citizens.

Healthcare organizations can improve their performance by assessing the quality of   doctor's services delivered to patients, quality of hospital services, patient's satisfaction level, cost of care and care outcomes.

References

1. *Quality of care: A Process for Making Strategic Choices in Health Systems.* World Health Organization. 2006.

2. Buttell, P., Handler, R., & Daley, J. (Aug, 2007). *Quality in Healthcare: Concepts and Practice.*

3. Hamidi, & Yadollah. (1 July, 2009). Strategic Leadership for Effectiveness of Quality Managers in Medical Sciences Universities: What Skill is Necessary? *Australian Journal of Basic and Applied Sciences.*

4. Altman, D.E., Clancy, C., & Blendon, R.J. (2004). Improving Patient Safety Five Years after the IOM Report. *N Engl J Med, 351,* 2041.

5. Bates, D.W., Cullen, D.J., & Laird, N. et al. (1995). Incidence of Adverse Drug Events and Potential Drug Events: Implications for Prevention. *JAMA, 247,* 29-34.

6. *Preventing Medication Errors.* Institute of Medicine Report. July, 2006, 1-4.

7. Huskins, W.C., Sonle, B.M., & O'Boyle, C. et al. (1998). Hospital Infection Prevention and Control: A Model of Improving the Quality of Hospital Care in Low and Middle Income Counties. *Infection Control and Hospital Epidemiology, 19,* 125-35.

8. *Joint Commission on Accreditation of Healthcare Organizations.* Comprehensive Accreditation Manuals for Hospitals. Oabrook Terrace, IL: Joint Commission on Accreditation of Healthcare Organizations, 2001.

9. Appropriateness in Health Care Delivery: Definitions, Measurement and Policy Implications. *Can Med Assoc J, 1996, 154,* 321-28.

10. Gumber, A. et al. (Apr-Jun, 2012). Declining Free Healthcare and Rising Treatment Costs in India- An Analysis of National Sample Surveys. 1986-2004. *Journal of Health Management, 14(2).*

11. Reddy, K.S., Patel, V., & Jha, P. et al. (2011). Towards Achievement of Universal Healthcare in India by 2020: A call to Action. The Lancet India Group for Universal Healthcare, *Lancet, 377,* 360-68.

MCQs

1. Which of the following statements is not true about quality?

a) A person perceives that quality is achieved even when he/she is not fully satisfied.
b) Quality means satisfying customer on a continuous basis.
c) Quality is dynamic in nature.
d) Quality requires improvements at regular intervals.

2. What are the three parameters used by Avedis Donabedian to define healthcare quality?

a) Facility, treatment and experience
b) System, diagnosis and satisfaction
c) Structure, process and outcome
d) None of the above

3. Which of the following is not the part of NABH's Patient Centered Standards?

a) Management of Medication (MOM)
b) Access, Assessment and Continuity of Care (ACC)
c) Hospital Infection Control (HIC)
d) Human Resource Management (HRM)

4. Which of the following is not the part of NABH's Organizational Centered Standards?

a) Continuous Quality Improvement (CQI)
b) Care of Patients (COP)
c) Information Management System (IMS)
d) Facility Management and Safety (FMS)

5. **WHO defines which of the following terms as the 'absence of preventable harm to a patient during the process of health care and reduction of risk of unnecessary harm associated with health care to an acceptable minimum'?**

   a) Quality

   b) Risk management

   c) Patient safety

   d) Patient care management

6. **What we call the infections that are acquired in the hospital by a patient in whom the infection was not present or incubating at the time of admission?**

   a) Adverse Drug Events

   b) Nosocomial Infections

   c) Medication Errors

   d) Surgical Complications

7. **Of the following adverse events, which is most common in India?**

   a) Hospital acquired infections

   b) Fall

   c) Medication errors

   d) None of the above

8. **What is a cross infection?**

   a) It is caused by patient's own endogenous flora.

   b) It is caused by a micro organism acquired from another person in the hospital.

   c) It is acquired from the substance recently contaminated from another human source.

   d) None of the above

9. **At which of the following stages about 50% of medication errors occur?**

   a) Dispensing of medicine stage

   b) Administration of medicine stage

   c) Transcribing of medicine stage

   d) Ordering of medicine stage

10. **Which of the following is true about Medical Asepsis?**

    a) It is known as sterile technique.

    b) It is known as clean technique.

    c) It is concerned with eliminating the spread of micro organisms through facility practices.

    d) Both (b) and (c)

11. **Which of the following is false about Surgical Asepsis?**

    a) It is a clean technique.

    b) It is the absence of all micro organisms within any type of invasive procedure.

    c) It aims to maintain a sterile field for surgery.

    d) It is a sterile technique.

12. **Which of the following is true about 'airborne transmission'?**

    a) It occurs when droplet nuclei < 5 micron in size are disseminated in air.

    b) Micro organisms can be acquired by direct contact, by contact with droplets over a distance up to 6 feet as well as by contact with objects recently contaminated with respiratory secretions.

    c) Diseases which are transmitted by this route include pneumonias, pertussis, diphtheria, influenza, mums, meningitis etc

    d) All of the above

13. What are the three globally applicable metrics for measuring the quality of care in hospital settings?

a) Consultation time, treatment prescribed, amount of money paid by patient.

b) Consultation time, number of questions asked, treatment prescribed.

c) Consultation time, number of questions asked, number of physical exams done.

d) Number of physical exams done, treatment prescribed, patient satisfaction.

14. How can 'know do gap' be defined in terms of healthcare?

a) It is a gap between the patient expectations and the actual treatment he/she receives.

b) It is a discrepancy between the prescribed medicine and the actual medicine given to a patient.

c) It is a gap between what the doctor can do and what he/she actually does in terms of treatment given to a patient.

d) None of the above

15. What among the following is not the area from which clinical indicators are chosen?

a) Patient assessment and care

b) Employee satisfaction indices

c) Infection control parameters

d) Surgical outcomes

16. What are the four major steps of PDSA cycle?

a) Prepare, Develop, Start, Action

b) Plan, Design, Simulate, Activate

c) Propose, Demonstrate, Start, Act

d) Plan, Do, Study, Act

17. Gap analysis is done to identify the gaps between the current state and the future state of an organization. It is a part of which of the following stages of strategic quality planning?

a) Strategy implementation stage

b) Strategy formulation stage

c) Strategy monitoring and evaluation stage

d) None of the above

Answer key

1. (a)   2. (c)   3. (d)   4. (b)   5. (c)   6. (b)   7. (a)   8. (b)
9. (d)   10. (d)   11. (a)   12. (a)   13. (c)   14. (c)   15. (b)   16. (d)
17. (b)

Chapter 4

Role of Informatics in Healthcare Delivery

Abstract

Informatics has revolutionalized the healthcare sector. Health information system helps in managing healthcare data with better efficiency. This chapter deals with health information system, its components, information security threats and the ways to prevent them.

Introduction

Information is defined as data with meaning. Informatics is the science of information. According to the U.S. National Library of Medicine, health informatics is the interdisciplinary study of design, development, adoption and application of IT based innovations in healthcare service delivery, management and planning.

Fundamental Theorem of Informatics

A person working in partnership with an information resource is 'better' than that same person unassisted. This theorem is applicable to healthcare also.

Information resource is any mechanism capable of providing information or knowledge or advice to support the person's ability to complete a task.

Health informatics in conjunction with health information technology can help clinicians in providing better healthcare.

Health information technology is the application of information processing involving both computer hardware and software that deals with the storage, retrieval, sharing and use of healthcare information, data and knowledge for communication and decision making.

Health information technology has tremendous potential to transform healthcare.

Many of the benefits of health IT include reduction of errors, elimination of redundant tests or better use of preventive services that can reduce future need for expensive services. All of these translate into financial benefits to patients in the form of lower bills as well as higher quality and more efficient care.

Health IT involves the development of health information system.

Health Information System

Health information system is an integrated system capable of capturing, storing, managing and exchanging health information of individuals and the data related to the activities of the healthcare organizations.

Following can be the components of a health information system-

1. **Electronic Medical Record (EMR) and Electronic Health Record (EHR)**

EMR is a repository of information regarding the health of a subject of care in computer processable form which is stored and transmitted securely and is accessible to multiple authorised users within one healthcare organisation.

EHR is an electronic record of health related information of an individual that conforms to nationally recognised interoperability standards and is accessible to authorised clinicians across more than one healthcare organization. EHRs build up a much broader picture of a patient's overall health by collecting information from all the clinicians involved in a patient's treatment.

EHRs facilitate the exchange of updated information in real time.

Following are the benefits of EMRs and EHRs-

(i) Both EMR and EHR help in reducing the number of medical errors and improve healthcare by keeping information accurate and up-to-date.

(ii) Duplicate testing can be reduced to save both patient's as well as provider's time.

(iii) More complete and updated patient information can lead to more accurate diagnoses and treatment.

(iv) Electronic reporting makes the patient's charts and documents much more clear.

2. Computerized Physician Order Entry (CPOE)

CPOE is an order entry application specifically designed to assist clinical practitioners in creating and managing medical orders for patient services and medications.

Following are the benefits of CPOE-

(i) Automated entry eliminates hand writing errors.

(ii) CPOE can reduce the time taken by an order to reach pharmacy.

(iii) CPOE can minimize errors that occur due to look alike, sound alike and spell alike drugs.

(iv) It is easy to interface CPOE with EHRs and decision support systems.

3. Clinical Decision Support System (CDSS)

CDSS provides assistance in clinical decision making tasks.

Following are the benefits of clinical decision support system-

(i) CDSS provides a list of possible disease diagnoses that relate to the patient's complaints.

(ii) CDSS gives guidelines for treatment related to specific diagnoses, recommends drug dosages and displays pop-ups for incompatible drugs.

(iii) CDSS helps in follow up management through reminder pop-ups for monitoring drug adverse events, for screening procedures such as mammography or for immunization.

(iv) It helps in deciding length of the hospital stay and minimizes the stay based on the patient's outcome.

(v) CDSS also alerts against duplicate testing.

4. Laboratory Information System

It manages and stores data for clinical laboratories. Benefits of using laboratory information system include tracking samples in real-time, managing logistics efficiently, eliminating human errors etc.

5. Policy and Procedure Management System (PPMS)

Policy and procedure management system can benefit the healthcare organization by centralizing all the policies and procedures at one location and by providing better collaboration between policy makers and followers. Policy and procedure management system helps to better comply with the policies.

6. Radiology Information System (RIS)

It manages medical imagery and associated data. Its functions include patient scheduling, resource management, examination performance tracking, reporting, results distribution and procedure billing.

7. Picture Archiving and Communication System (PACS)

It is used to securely store and digitally transmit electronic images and clinically relevant reports. This system provides digital images that can be zoomed for a closer look. The images can be manipulated for better viewing and analysis. Other benefits of PACS include improved data management, easy access to patient's reports and images, chronological data management etc.

8. Tele-health and other Remote Patient Monitoring Technology (Telemedicine)

Tele-health involves the use of tele-communications and virtual technology to deliver healthcare. It broadly applies to both clinical and non-clinical settings. Tele-health also includes provider training, administrative meetings, continuing medical education etc.

Tele-medicine specifically refers to remote clinical services. Tele-medicine programs most frequently provide evaluation, diagnoses or prescriptive services to the patients.

9. Administrative, Billing and Financial Systems

These systems help in smooth functioning of administrative services, bringing transparency in billing services and improving financial performance of the healthcare organizations.

Electronic Health Records

According to studies reported on Health IT.gov, the majority of physicians believe that electronic health records provide a better view of their patient's total health, allowing for better diagnosis while reducing the chance of medical errors. Physicians also cite improved efficiency within their practices, which in turn translates into an enhanced patient experience.

Cloud-based EHR

Cloud based EHR maintains health files in the cloud rather than on internal servers located at a medical facility. It is the responsibility of the cloud based service providers to make sure that the patient's files are kept confidential and protected. Benefits of cloud based EHR include faster deployment, cost flexibility, easy accessibility and greater security.

Client-Server EHR

In a client server EHR, end users such as physicians or nurses use software on their computers to access data which is centralized and hosted internally.

EHR Vendors

Top EHR vendors include Epic, Cerner, athenahealth, eClinicalWorks, Allscripts, Practice Fusion, AdvancedMD etc. The selection of an EHR vendor is said to be successful only when it suits the EHR needs of an organization.

According to a report by Heather Landi dated May 25, 2018, Epic and Cerner continue to maintain the largest EMR market share among small hospitals (with 200 or fewer beds), with 26.7% market share and 24.8% respectively. Unlike EMRs, EHRs are designed to share information with other healthcare providers. So, an EHR needs to be highly inter-operable.

One of the main issues EHR vendors face is lack of consistency between systems and inability to customize capabilities, especially in platforms by Epic and Cerner. Inconsistency in data categorization and locations can lead to difficulty in data sharing and communication between facilities with differing platforms.

In the year 1992, Epic released the first Windows based EMR called EpicCare which is now known as EpicCare Ambulatory and is used in outpatient settings. Epic runs on a 47 years old programming language called MUMPS, which makes it incompatible to interface with software from other companies for consolidating patient data. Critics claim that Epic is not inter-operable due to vendor locking.

According to the KLAS report, EpicCare Ambulatory EHR is preferred by only 24% of 26 to 100 physician group while eClinicalWorks EHR is preferred by 51% of 26 to 100 physician group.

eClinicalWorks V11 EHR is a 2015 Edition Certified product under the ONC Health IT Certification Program. It has the features like EVA (eClinicalWorks Virtual Assistant), Available anytime, anywhere, on any device, In place editing, Patient safety and compliance dashboards, Free interoperability through CommonWell and Carequality and Enhanced prescribing of controlled substances.

According to a report published by Healthcare IT News, as far as physician's satisfaction is concerned eClinicalWorks and athenahealth score big in ambulatory settings. KLAS report suggests, athenahealth's product athenaClinicals is preferred by 35% of 26 to 100 physician group.

athenaClinicals is a cloud based EHR which was launched in 2006. It has the features like Focus on patients, Easy interoperability, Clinical efficiency, Automated workflows, Faster documentation and Easy attestation. athenaClinicals has been ranked as leading the market in EHR usability, due to its productivity and ability to reduce provider's work, effectiveness of delivering patient care, and intuitive user interface. eClinicalWorks and athenahealth would be a good fit for an organization which has the following set of criteria-

(i)   EHR system founded within past 20 Years

(ii) Facility capacity = over 200 beds

(iii) Physicians = 26-100

(iv) Ease of use, the most important feature

Clinical Decision Support System (CDSS)

It is an application that analyses data to help healthcare providers make decisions during patient care. There are two main types of clinical decision support system.

(i)   Knowledge based CDSS-

It uses a knowledge base, applies rules to patient's data using an inference engine and then displays the results.

(ii) Non-knowledge based CDSS-

It relies on machine learning to analyse clinical data.

Push and Pull solutions for CDSS

Push and Pull solutions are implemented as part of a successful clinical decision support strategy.

Push solution automatically delivers what is specifically needed to the user e.g. automatic order sets and critical care pathways.

Pull solution requires voluntary engagement. It allows providers to seek and find current, credible, evidence based information to guide care e.g. on demand reference solutions and info buttons.

Following points should be considered while choosing push and pull solutions for clinical decision support system-

(i) Information should be presented at the time it is needed, which is usually when a decision has to be made e.g. a drug dosage information is best to be available at the time the doctor is prescribing medicines.

(ii) New information should be presented when it arrives, especially if information would influence the clinician's decision e.g. if the report form monitoring drug level in a patient's blood shows the patient has too much of a prescribed medication in his or her system, the physician might need to take immediate action based on that information. In this case, information should be brought to their attention with a push alert.

(iii) Information should reach the clinician to stop a dangerous decision so that the harm to a patient can be avoided e.g. if the physician has just ordered a drug that the patient is allergic to, warning should be presented before the order goes through in a push alert.

(iv) It is important to monitor the frequency of presentation of information. Too frequent repetition of similar information can tend to get ignored. Frequent repetition can lead to alarm fatigue. Alarm fatigue is a sensory overload where clinicians are exposed to an excessive number of alarms which can result in desensitization to alarms. Patient's deaths have been attributed to alarm fatigue.

Health Information Exchange

Health Information exchange allows healthcare professionals and patients to appropriately access and securely share patient's medical information electronically. It results in improving the speed, quality, safety and cost of patient care. Timely sharing of vital patient's information leads to better decision making at the point of care and helps healthcare providers to avoid readmissions, avoid medication errors, improve diagnoses and decrease duplicate testing.

Following are key components of health information exchange infrastructure-

1. Master Patient Index

2. Document Registry

3. Document / Image Repository

Consider the following example to understand the working of health information exchange-

When a primary care physician treats the patient, a summary containing the clinical information is created. This document is published into the 'central document repository' and the existence of the document is simultaneously registered with a pointer to its location in the 'document registry.' The data has thereby been published from the primary care physician's EMR into the health information exchange where it can be queried by users at other organizations such as specialty practice with appropriate authorization to view the patient's clinical information.

To retrieve the clinical data related to a patient whose information has been published into the health information exchange by a primary care physician, the specialty practice send a query into the patient ID manager as an initial step to see if the patient exists in the health information exchange.

When confirmation is received, the specialty practice then sends a query to the document registry to see if there are any clinical documents for the patient. If a list of documents return, specialty practice from that list, can then query directly to the document repository for a primary care physician via the pointer and open the specific document. The process starts over when the specialty practice publishes a document into the health information exchange following the patient's visit.

Forms of Health Information Exchange-

1. Directed Exchange

It is used by healthcare providers to easily and securely send patient's information such as laboratory orders and results, patient referrals or discharge summaries directly to another healthcare professional. This information is sent over the internet in an encrypted, secure and reliable manner. e.g. a primary care provider can directly send electronic care summaries that include medications, problems and lab results to a specialist when referring their patients. This information helps to inform the visit and prevents the duplication of tests, redundant collection of information from the patient and medication errors.

Directed exchange can also be used for sending immunization data to public health organizations.

2. Query based Exchange

It is used by healthcare providers to search and discover accessible clinical sources on a patient. They find or request information on a patient from other healthcare providers. This type of exchange is often used when delivering unplanned care.

e.g. emergency room physicians who can utilize query based exchange to access patient information such as medications, recent radiology images, problem lists etc might adjust treatment plans to avoid adverse medication reactions or duplicate testing.

3. Consumer mediated Exchange

It provides patients with access to their health information, allowing them to manage their healthcare online.

Patients can directly participate in their care coordination by-

    a) Providing their health information to other healthcare providers.

    b) Identifying and correcting wrong or missing health information.

    c) Identifying and correcting incorrect billing information.

    d) Tracking and monitoring their own health.

Data Standards

In order to function properly, systems that exchange information must agree to certain data standards. Data standards are the rules to describe how the data is recovered to ensure consistency across multiple sources.

Following are the categories of data standards-

1. Vocabulary Standards

These are the standardized nomenclatures and code sets used to describe clinical problems and procedures, medications and allergies.

2. Content Exchange Standards

These are the standards used to share clinical information such as clinical summaries and prescriptions using structured electronic documents.

3. Privacy and Security Standards

These standards relate to authentication, access control and transmission security.

Privacy and security standards may define for how files are physically stored on hardware storage devices to ensure that inappropriate tampering with the storage device cannot be used to steal private healthcare data.

In India, the Ministry of Health and Family Welfare has set up an Integrated Health Information Platform (IHIP) with the aim to introduce a 'uniform system' for maintenance and exchange of electronic medical records by the hospitals and healthcare providers.

Privacy, Security and Confidentiality Issues

1. Privacy

Privacy is the individual's right to keep information to himself or herself.

2. Confidentiality

Confidentiality is the individual's right to keep information about himself or herself from being disclosed to other people. When a patient vests confidentiality in a physician and a healthcare system, it is expected that personal information is kept confidential and not disclosed to others.

3. Security

Security is the activity of protecting personal information. Security should address the physical security of the building, equipment and storage media as well as the data and informational assets retained by all healthcare organizations.

Security Threats

Security threat is a malicious attack that aims to corrupt or steal data or disrupt an organization's systems.

Following are the common types of informational security threats-

1. Insider Threats

Insider threat occurs when individuals closely associated with an organization and having authorized access to its network, intentionally or unintentially misuse that access to negatively affect the organization's critical data or systems. There are three main types of insider threats.

(i) Compromised Users

These are the outsiders who access information under the credentials of a legitimate user e.g. if the employee of an organization grants access to the attacker by clicking on phishing link in an email.

(ii) Careless Users

They don't strictly comply with the organization's business rules and policies e.g. if an employee shares login information with others.

(iii) Malicious Users

They intentionally elude cyber security protocols to delete data, steal data or share it with others. Since malicious users are involved in the attack, they can cover up their tracks. It makes detection even more difficult.

Following are the ways to prevent insider threats-

(i) Limit employees' access to only those resources which are needed to perform their jobs.

(ii) Train new employees on security awareness before allowing them to access the network.

(iii) Set up contractors and other free lancers with temporary accounts that expire on specific dates such as the dates at which their contracts end.

(iv) Implement two factor authentication that requires each user to provide a second piece of identifying information in addition to a password.

(v) Install employee monitoring software to help reduce the risk of data breach and the theft of intellectual property.

2. Viruses and Worms

Computer virus is a malicious code that replicates by copying itself to another program, system or host file. Virus must be triggered by the activation of its host. Program, software or executable file can act as a host for the virus. Viruses need human intervention to spread.

Worm is a standalone malicious program that can self-replicate and propagate independently as soon as it breaches the system.

Following are the ways to prevent viruses and worms-

(i) Install antivirus and antimalware software on all systems and networked devices.

(ii) Train users not to download attachments or click on links in emails from unknown senders.

(iii) Avoid downloading free software from untrusted websites.

3. Botnets

Botnet is a collection of internet connected devices, including PCs, mobile devices, servers and IOT devices that are infected and remotely controlled by a common type of malware. These infected devices can be used to send email spam, engage in click fraud campaigns and generate malicious traffic for distributed denial-of-service attacks.

Following are the ways to prevent botnets-

(i) Monitor network performance and activity to detect any irregular network behaviour.

(ii) Keep the operating system up to date.

(iii) Keep all software up to date

(iv) Implement anti-botnet tools.

4. Phishing

Phishing is the fraudulent attempt to obtain sensitive information such as usernames, passwords and credit card details by disguising oneself as a trustworthy entity. In most cases, hackers send out fake emails that look as if they are coming from legitimate sources. They ask the users to take some recommended action such as clicking on links in emails that take them to fraudulent websites that ask for personal information or install malware on their devices.

Following are the ways to prevent phishing-

(i) Don't click on links in emails from unknown senders.

(ii) Avoid downloading free software from untrusted websites.

5. Distributed denial-of-service attacks

In a distributed denial-of-service attack, multiple compromised machines attack a target, such as a server, website or other network resource, making the target totally inoperable.

Following are the ways to prevent distributed denial-of-service attacks-

(i) Implement technology to monitor networks visually and know how much bandwidth a site uses on an average.

(ii) Ensure servers have the capacity to handle heavy traffic spikes and to address security problems.

(iii) Update and patch firewalls and network security programs.

6. Advanced Persistent Threat (APT) attacks

In such attacks, an unauthorised intruder penetrates a network and remains undetected for an extended period of time. Rather than causing damage to a system or network, the goal of an APT attack is to monitor network activity and steal information. Cyber criminals use APT attacks to target large enterprises and National states to steal data over a long period.

Following are the ways to prevent APT attacks-

(i) Deploy software, hardware or cloud firewall to guard against APT attacks.

(ii) Use web application firewall to detect and prevent attacks coming from web applications by inspecting HTTP traffic.

7. Ransomware

In a ransomware attack, the victim's computer is locked typically by encryption, which keeps him/her away from using the device or data stored in it. To regain access to the device or data, the victim has to pay the hacker a ransom.

Following are the ways to prevent ransomware attacks-

(i) User should regularly back up their computing devices and update all software including anti-virus software.

(ii) User should avoid clicking on links in emails or opening email attachments from unknown sources.

(iii) Organizations should couple a traditional firewall that blocks unauthorized access to computer or networks with a program that filters web content and focuses on sites that may introduce malware.

8. Malvertising

It is a technique used by cyber criminals to inject malicious code into legitimate online advertising networks and web pages. This code typically redirects users to malicious websites or installs malware on their computers or mobile devices.

Following are the ways to prevent malvertising-

(i) Ad networks should add validation which can reduce the chances for user to be compromised.

(ii) Web hosts should periodically check their websites from an unpatched system and monitor that system to detect any malicious activity.

Generic Ways to Prevent IT Security Threats

1. Use strong authentication to verify the identity of a user or a device. It may be a single factor authentication like biometrics authentication, two factor authentication like user provided username, password (knowledge factor) and one time password (possession factor) or multi factor authentication like user provided physical token, password in conjunction with biometric data. Allow only authorized users to access the resources of an organization.

2. Deploy integrity management solutions to assess and maintain soundness of the overall system.

3. Use digital signatures to validate the identity of the sender.

4. Use firewalls for network security.

5. Install security software tools like anti-malware, anti-spyware, anti-virus software, password managers, encryption software etc.

Population Health Informatics

It is the systematic application of health IT and other digital technologies and information sciences for the improvement of health and wellbeing of a defined community or target population.

Public Health Informatics

It is the application of informatics in areas of public health, including surveillance, prevention, preparedness and health promotion.

Public health informatics focuses on those aspects of public health that enable the development and use of interoperable information systems for public health functions such as bio surveillance outbreak management, electronic laboratory reporting and prevention.

Global Health Informatics

It is a growing multi-disciplinary field that combines research methods and applications of technology to improve healthcare systems and outcomes.

Conclusion

Healthcare systems are facing many challenges including growing population, increasing complexity of care services and limited resources to deliver services. These challenges require more innovative approaches to provide healthcare services to large number of people.

It is challenging to implement information technology in Indian healthcare sector. In India, there is no comprehensive policy on health information technology. It results in lack of clarity on health IT standards and guidelines. Most of the staff working in Indian healthcare organizations has limited knowledge of computers which is not sufficient enough to implement health IT solutions. Also some of the healthcare organizations cannot afford the high cost needed in health IT infrastructure deployment.

In order to promote the use of health information technology, the government should provide funding to the healthcare organizations. It will help them in improving current infrastructure, purchasing and installing new technology, training existing staff and recruiting competent health staff.

References

1. Williams, C., Mostashari, F., & Mertz K. et al. (2012). From the Office of the National Coordinator: The Strategy for Advancing the Exchange of Health Information. *Health Affairs, 31(3)*, 527-36.

2. Retrieved from

    https://www.healthit.gov/topic/health-it-and-health-information-exchange-basics/what-hie.

3. Retrieved from
   https://www.hhmglobal.com/knowledge-bank/articles/how-to-push-and-pull-your-way-to-a-successful-clinical-decision-support-strategy.

4. *HIMMS Dictionary of Healthcare Information Technology Terms, Acronyms and Organizations,* 2nd Edition, 2010, Appendix B, p.190.

5. American Academy of Family Physicians (AAFP), Center for Health IT, 2013.

6. *HIMMS Dictionary of Healthcare Information Technology Terms, Acronyms and Organizations,* 3rd Edition, 2013, p.75.

7. *Report on Uniform Data Standards for Patient Medical Record Information.* National Committee on Vital and Health Statistics (NCVHS). July 6, 2000, 21-22.

8. *IEEE Standard Computer Dictionary: A Compilation of IEEE Standard Computer Glossaries.* Institute of Electrical and Electronics Engineers. New York, 1990.

9. Retrieved from
   https://www.google.com/amp/s/searchsecurity.techtarget.com/feature/Top-10-types-of-information-security-threats-for-IT-terms%3famp=1.

10. Retrieved from
    https://www.google.com/amp/s/searchsecurity.techtarget.com/definition/two-factor-authentication%3famp=1.

MCQs

1. According to the U.S. National Library of Medicine, which of the following is the correct definition of Health Informatics?

a) It is defined as meaningful healthcare data.

b) It is the interdisciplinary study of design, development, adoption and application of IT based innovations in healthcare service delivery, management and planning.

c) It is the science of healthcare information.

d) None of the above

2. What is the fundamental theorem of Informatics?

a) Informatics in conjunction with information technology gives better results.

b) Human resource is better than the AI assisted system.

c) A person working in partnership with an information resource is better than that same person unassisted.

d) None of the above

3. Which of the following is an integrated system capable of capturing, storing, managing and exchanging health information of individuals and the data related to the activities of the healthcare organizations?

a) Health Information System

b) Health Informatics

c) Health Information Technology

d) None of the above

4. Which of the following statements is false about Electronic Health Record (EHR)?

a) The health information in EHR conforms to nationally recognized interoperability standards.

b) The information in EHR is accessible to multiple authorized users within one healthcare organization.

c) EHR collects information from all the clinicians involved in a patient's treatment.

d) EHR facilitates the exchange of updated information in real time.

5. Which of the following is not the component of a Health Information System?

a) Electronic Health Record

b) Clinical Decision Support System

c) Radiology Information System

d) Botnets

6. **Which of the following is specifically designed to assist clinical practitioners in creating and managing medical orders for patient services and medications?**

   a) Centralized patient order entry

   b) Centralized prescription order entry

   c) Clinical practitioner order entry

   d) Computerized physician order entry

7. **Which of the following statements is false about Clinical Decision Support System?**

   a) It provides a list of possible disease diagnoses related to the patient's complaints.

   b) It gives guidelines for treatments related to specific diagnoses and recommends drug dosages.

   c) It reduces the time taken by the order to reach pharmacy.

   d) It helps in monitoring drug adverse events.

8. **Which of the following systems centralizes all the policies and procedures at one location and provides better collaboration between policy makers and followers?**

   a) Picture Archiving and Communication System

   b) Policy and Procedure Management System

   c) Central Policy System

   d) Policy Collaboration System

9. **Which of the following is a benefit of Picture Archiving and Communication System?**

   a) It securely stores and digitally transmits electronic images and clinically relevant reports.

   b) It provides digital images that can be zoomed for a closer look.

   c) The images provided by it can be manipulated for better viewing and analysis.

   d) All of the above

10. What an EHR must have in order to share information with other healthcare providers smoothly?

a) User friendly

b) Inter operability

c) Consistency

d) Customizing capabilities

11. Which of the following statements is false about 'pull' solution for clinical decision support system?

a) It allows healthcare providers to seek and find current, credible evidence based information to guide care.

b) It requires voluntary engagement.

c) Automatic order sets is an example of pull solution.

d) Info buttons is an example of pull solution.

12. Which of the following statements is false about Directed Health Information Exchange?

a) It is used by healthcare providers to send patient's information directly to another healthcare professional.

b) The information is sent over the internet in an encrypted, secure and reliable manner.

c) It allows patients to manage their healthcare online.

d) It can be used for sending immunization data to public health organizations.

13. Which of the following are the standardized nomenclatures and code sets used to describe clinical problems and procedures, medications and allergies?

a) Content exchange standards

b) Privacy and security standards

c) Text standards

d) Vocabulary standards

14. **If the patient does not want to tell the doctor that he/she dropped out of college years ago, then this is an example of which of the following?**

    a) Privacy

    b) Confidentiality

    c) Security

    d) The common good

15. **Which of the following users intentionally elude cyber security protocols to delete data, steal data or share it with others?**

    a) Compromised users

    b) Careless users

    c) Smart users

    d) Malicious users

16. **Which of the following statements is false about a computer virus?**

    a) It is a malicious code that replicates by copying itself to another program, system or host file.

    b) Virus must be triggered by the activation of its host.

    c) Viruses need human intervention to spread.

    d) None of the above

17. **Which of the following is a fraudulent attempt to obtain sensitive information such as usernames, passwords etc by disguising oneself as a trust worthy entity?**

    a) Distributed denial-of-service attack

    b) Advanced Persistent Threat attack

    c) Phishing

    d) Botnet

18. In which of the following attacks, an unauthorized intruder penetrates a network and remains undetected for an extended period of time?

a) Advanced Persistent Threat attack

b) Distributed denial-of-service attack

c) Phishing

d) None of the above

19. In which of the following a malicious code is injected into legitimate online advertising networks and web pages?

a) Ransomware

b) Malvertising

c) Phishing

d) Mal networking

20. How can population health informatics be defined?

a) It is the application of informatics for the improvement of health of a defined community.

b) It is a multi-disciplinary field that combines research methods and applications of technology to improve healthcare systems and outcomes.

c) It is the application of informatics in areas of public health including surveillance, prevention, preparedness and health promotion.

d) None of the above

Answer key

1. (b)   2. (c)   3. (a)   4. (b)   5. (d)   6. (d)   7. (c)   8. (b)

9. (d)   10. (b)   11. (c)   12. (c)   13. (d)   14. (a)   15. (d)   16. (d)

17. (c)   18. (a)   19. (b)   20. (a)

Chapter 5

Telemedicine: An Emerging Trend in Healthcare Technology

Abstract

Telemedicine is remote diagnosis and treatment of patients by means of telecommunications technology. It holds a great potential to improve the quality, access and affordability of healthcare. This chapter analyzes the contribution of both public and private sector in making telemedicine an alternate way of providing healthcare services especially in rural India.

Introduction

Telemedicine has gained tremendous popularity in developing countries where rural population is deprived of even basic healthcare. Telemedicine market has witnessed spectacular growth mainly because of convergence of Information Technology Communication and Healthcare.

Telemedicine may be as simple as two health professionals discussing a case over the telephone or as complex as using satellite technology and video conferencing equipment to conduct a real time consultation between medical specialists in two different countries.

India faces a great challenge of providing affordable healthcare to all. About 70% of the total population lives in rural areas. Healthcare system in these areas has to cope with lot of problems like severe shortage of healthcare professionals, lack of medical facilities, basic infrastructure etc. About 60-80 % of the physician positions in different specialties are vacant in rural healthcare services. According to a study conducted in 2009 by the Indian Medical Society, 75% of the qualified consulting doctors in India reside in urban areas, 23% in semi-urban areas and only 2% in rural areas. In such a scenario, telemedicine can play a pivotal role in providing healthcare services to rural population of India.

Using a number of high speed satellite and terrestrial telecommunication links, centralization and coordination of resources and support of government, it has been possible to reach and access the Indian population spread out in heterogeneous geography and thus achieve the goal of health for all. However, all the activities must be evaluated in a national framework and many areas, such as national e-health policy and legal/ethical issues need to be addressed.

Telemedicine in India

Telemedicine aims at providing technology based primary healthcare services at minimal costs in those parts of India where basic medical facilities are not easily accessible.

There are two types of technology used in telemedicine.

The first is Asynchronous type technology in which pre recorded data is exchanged between two or more individuals at different times and locations. This technology is also called 'store and forward'. Digital camera is used to take digital images which are stored and then forwarded to another location by a computer. This technology is used in tele-radiology, tele pathology, tele dermatology etc.

The other is Synchronous type technology in which real time data is exchanged. The patient or the telemedicine coordinator is at one site and the specialist at the referral site. Both the locations are equipped with video conferencing facility that allows a real time consultation to take place. This technology is preferred in psychiatry, internal medicine, pediatrics, cardiology, obstetrics and gynaecology, neurology etc.

In India, the first telemedicine pilot project was started by ISRO in collaboration with Apollo Hospitals Group in 2001, under which a telemedicine link was established between an Apollo rural hospital at Aragonda village in the Chittor district of Andhra Pradesh and the Apollo hospital at Chennai. ISRO provided the necessary communication links via its INSAT satellites while Apollo group equipped their hospitals with desired medical infrastructure.

Since then various government agencies like Department of Information Technology and Ministry of Health and Family Welfare, State governments, Premier medical and technical institutions, Private hospitals and Companies of India have taken several initiatives with the aim of providing quality healthcare facilities to rural and remote parts of the country.

Telemedicine service providers have to deal with many complex issues like availability of technology at reasonable cost, interruption in power supply, lack of trained manpower, availability of funds, data privacy and security concerns.

Telemedicine has many advantages associated with it. Telemedicine eliminates distance barriers and improves access to quality health services for the population living in underserved areas. It is also helpful in critical care situations where moving a patient is undesirable or not feasible.

Around 40% of Indian households report of having borrowed or sold assets to pay for hospitalization expenditure. For rural population paying out of pocket for healthcare is a major burden. Telemedicine can bring some relief to them. Tele-education and tele CME upgrade the knowledge of the rural physicians.

Indian Space Research Organization (ISRO)

ISRO has deployed a SATCOM based telemedicine network across the country. It has started a telemedicine program in 2001 with the aim to connect remote, rural healthcare providers to major specialty hospitals in cities and towns through the Indian satellites. The states and regions that are covered under this program include Jammu & Kashmir, Ladakh, Andaman & Nicobar Islands, Lakshdweep Islands, North Eastern States, tribal districts of Kerala, Karnataka, Chattisgarh, Punjab, West Bengal, Odisha, Andhra Pradesh, Maharashtra, Jharkhand and Rajasthan. Presently, the telemedicine network of ISRO covers about 384 hospitals with 60 specialty hospitals connected to 306 remote/rural/district/medical college hospitals and 18 mobile telemedicine units.

ISRO's Model of Telemedicine

ISRO uses a multi-point to multi-point system. Computers at a specialty hospital connect to a common terminal which links via satellite to rural district hospitals and clinics that have ISRO connectivity in space. To build an ISRO terminal, medical centers have to pay a substantial up-front-cost (around 6,00,000 INR). But once built, the ISRO network is provided as a free service for hospitals that are linked to rural telemedicine centers.

In 2001, ISRO, Department of Space (DOS) and the North Eastern Council (NEC) collaborated to establish North Eastern Space Applications Centre (NESAC). NESAC started an ISRO-NEC telemedicine project in 2004 utilizing satellite communication through very small aperture terminal (VSAT). They formulated a plan to commission 72 telemedicine regional nodal centers in all districts of north eastern states like Assam, Arunachal Pradesh, Manipur, Mizoram, Meghalaya, Nagaland, Tripura and Sikkim. Around 25 regional telemedicine centers have been commissioned and remaining 47 are in various stages of implementation.

Another telemedicine project known as Army Telemedicine Network for NER is also operational in the north eastern states in collaboration with Indian Army from March 2008. Under this network a total of 6 telemedicine centers have been commissioned in various army hospitals in the north eastern region.

Tripura, one of the north eastern states of India, has set an example of successful implementation of telemedicine program in the country. In Tripura, telemedicine set up has been implemented at 27 hospitals including 3 referral hospitals and 24 nodal hospitals. All these centers are interconnected with internet speeds of 512Kbps/2Mbps for data transfer and data management. This project has been successful in treating approximately 1,16,376 patients by telemedicine from June 2009 to 31st December 2017.

Some of the other successful telemedicine pilot projects in which ISRO played a key role include telemedicine network in West Bengal for diagnosis and monitoring of tropical diseases, the oncology network in Kerala and Tamil Nadu, the network of specialty healthcare access in rural areas of Punjab, Maharashtra and Himachal Pradesh.

Role of Indian Government in Promoting Telemedicine

Following table shows the initiatives taken by Ministry of Health and Family Welfare, Government of India to promote telemedicine for catering healthcare needs of rural population of India-

2003	Defined National standards on telemedicine.
2005	Constituted National steering committee on telemedicine.
(2007-2012) 11th Five Year Plan	In 11th Five Year Plan, there was a budget Head by Planning Commission for e-Health including telemedicine.
2007	Established National Rural Telemedicine Network. It includes: 1. Designing, development and implementation of low cost rural telemedicine infrastructure. 2. Establishment of village tele-ambulance system and rural emergency healthcare services/ trauma care module. 3. Development of Rural Health Knowledge Resource through web portal and e-CME module. 4. Providing technology platform for harvest, compilation, storage (data base) at Regional District Hub and Central Data Centre at Ministry of Health and Family Welfare, archive and distribution across network. 5. Released grants to all states/UTs for National Rural Telemedicine Network.

(2012-2017) 12th Five Year Plan	Formulated strategy for ICT applications in healthcare. It includes: 1. Access to CME (continuing medical education) and skill up-gradation programs as well as backup support on telemedicine. 2. Deployment of country wide Hospital Management Information System (HMIS). 3. Use of ICT in health education, public health status analysis and expansion of health related research. 4. Introducing m-Health which involves use of mobile phones to speed up transmission. 5. Allocated funds for e-health including telemedicine.
2013	1. All Regional Cancer Centers along with four peripheral hospitals at district level were networked under OncoNet project. 2. Deployed Tele-ophthalmology projects in most of the states empowering vision centers to link Expert Eye Centers. 3. Proposed a 'National Medical College Network' project to link Government medical colleges having National Knowledge Network connectivity. 4. Started pilot projects at three sites under National Optical Fiber Network Initiative.
2015	Launched a telemedicine initiative in collaboration with Apollo Hospitals. As part of the service named 'Sehat', people in rural areas can consult doctors through video link and can also online order generic drugs.

2016	1. Signed a Memorandum of Understanding (MoU) with ISRO to expand its telemedicine network to remote places.
	2. Approved Centrally Sponsored Scheme (CSS) for establishment of National Medical College Network (NMCN), wherein 41 Government Medical Colleges are being networked in the first phase riding over National Knowledge Network- high speed bandwidth connectivity, with the purpose of e-Education and e-Healthcare delivery.
	3. Proposed setting up of new Telemedicine nodes in collaboration with ISRO at the following remote locations- (i) One district each in Himachal Pradesh, Odisha, Arunachal Pradesh and Meghalaya. (ii) Chardhams, Kailash Mansarovar, Amarnath and Ayappa pilgrimage places.
	4. Extended financial and technical support to state governments for strengthening & promoting Telemedicine network under their respective States/ Union Territories Programme Implementation Plan (PIPs) of National Health Mission (NHM) scheme.

Department of Information Technology (DIT), Government of India plays a leading role in the implementation of telemedicine initiatives in India. It creates manual of standards, best practices and procedures to govern the delivery of healthcare. It provides funds for the development of various software systems to support its network of clinics.

Medical Institutions of India have also taken steps to spread telemedicine network. All India Institute of Medical Sciences, New Delhi is linked with hospitals in Jammu and Kashmir, Haryana, Odisha and north eastern states while Postgraduate Institute of Medical Education and Research,

Chandigarh, is linked with district hospitals of Punjab and Himachal States. Both institutes are considered as leaders in telemedicine programming and dissemination. The School of Telemedicine and Biomedical Informatics has been established by the Sanjay Gandhi Postgraduate Institute of Medical Sciences, Lucknow with the financial support of the Government of Uttar Pradesh and the Department of Information Technology, Ministry of Communication & IT, Government of India. It is the National Resource Centre for telemedicine.

In the corporate sector, some of the major telemedicine players are Apollo Hospitals Group, World Health Partners, Narayana Health, Sankara Nethralaya etc.

Apollo Hospitals Group

It established Apollo Telemedicine Networking Foundation (ATNF) in 1999 with the aim of giving remote consultation and second opinion to both patients and doctors for whom access to quality healthcare is difficult due to distance and spiraling costs.

Today, ATNF has emerged as India's single largest turnkey provider in the area of telemedicine with over 150 telemedicine centers across the globe.

The Apollo Telemedicine Centers comprise of a Telemedicine Specialty Centre (TSC) and a Telemedicine Consultation Centre (TCC). TSCs are set up at the Apollo Multi Specialty Hospitals in cities like Chennai, Hyderabad, Delhi, Bangalore, Kolkata etc, where experts from different fields are available for consultation. TCCs are set up in peripheral centers from where the technician and patient can consult the specialist located at TSC. One of the essential devices used for consultation is a video conferencing tool accompanied by a voice transmission enabler that is connected to ISDN lines and to the TV both at TSC and TCC. From the consultation center, X-rays, CT scan, Color Doppler, ultra sound etc can be transferred over the ISDN line or IP with the help of an interface. In Telemedicine Specialty Centre, medical records are received on the system and can alternatively be viewed on the TV using an interface. In the absence of high definition video conferencing camera, a high definition web camera can also be used between TSC and TCC. For better transmission of X-rays and echo-cardiograms, a high resolution/ luminosity sub system is used that enables ECG readings to be seen at the TSC. An electronic or digital stethoscope is used to hear heart beats. The equipment is placed on the patient and connected to the telephone line and the doctor at TSC can hear heart beats on the system. In case of video conferencing, the voice is transferred using a voice enabling instrument attached to video conferencing camera. It has features like echo-canceller and noise reduction units for better transmission of heart sounds etc.

Apollo Telemedicine Networking Foundation's web enabled Telemedicine Application 'Medintegra WEB' supports the platform to carry out telemedicine consultation. The software collects the patient's data and converts it into a secure and confidential Electronic Medical Record (EMR). This data is then transferred to TSC where authorized specialist studies it and based on the investigation gives his/her expert opinion which is transmitted back to TCC. Apollo Telehealth services include Tele Clinics, Tele Radiology, Tele Cardiology, Tele Dermatology, Tele Pathology, Tele Emergency, Remote Condition Management Programs, Mobile Telemedicine Units, Tele Healthcare, Tele Education and Tele ICU (I-SEE-U facility that enables virtual visits to ICU).

In 2013, Apollo Hospitals started an initiative 'Telemedicine 2.0' with the aim of integrating healthcare delivery model with new age technology. Under this initiative, Telehealth services are provided on mobile phones and tablets to make tele health more user friendly.

In 2015, Apollo Hospitals set up one of the highest telemedicine stations in the world, under the government assisted Himachal Pradesh Telehealth Services Project.

World Health Partners (WHP)

WHP does not have its own network of telemedicine clinics. It coordinates a network of entrepreneurs' independent clinics. The main advantage of such type of franchise service model is that the local franchisees better understand the dynamics, needs and issues specific to their villages.

WHP has over 12,000 'Sky Centers' run by local entrepreneurs located in the remotest areas of Bihar and Uttar Pradesh. At these centers, WHP's 'ALTHEA' system is used. A specially developed application is loaded on a laptop or tablet and is used as a platform to integrate commonly available, medically certified diagnostic devices. The system currently uses devices to measure blood pressure, pulse, temperature, blood sugar, blood count, foetal sounds, and cardiac signals with provision for adding otoscope for ear examination and dermascope for skin. The system can work in any digital environment ranging from 2G to 3G, 4G and internet. The village facilitator uses pre-coded checkboxes in English or in local languages, so writing text is completely eliminated. An algorithm combines the symptoms registered by a village user with basic vital parameters and patient history to generate a list of differential diagnosis for the doctor. The system allows automatic generation of a list of most probable investigations and medicines for each diagnosis which will enable the doctor to quickly select his/her choices and doses. In case the doctor wants to overrule the differential diagnosis suggested by the system, he/she can access the entire 'International Classification of Diseases' latest version of the World Health Organization. The system also provides task lists for predictable services such as estimation of gestational age, growth monitoring and immunization. Each interaction between a tele healthcare seeker and provider is captured and stored in the internet cloud as an Electronic Medical Record (EMR) under a unique patient identity which makes referrals easier. The ALTHEA system can transmit live videos and audios in real time with the bandwidth strength of 40 Kbps making it suitable even in a 2G environment.

Narayana Health

In 2016, a Memorandum of Understanding (MoU) was signed between Narayana Health and CISCO. According to it, both the parties dedicated themselves to deliver affordable healthcare services remotely using CISCO's Virtual Expertise Digital Solution. This solution enables real time telemetry of medical device data, audio, high definition two way video, ECG and other vitals and radiology, analytics of medical reports and a web based portal which supports mobile end points. Detailed examination of a patient can be possible now with the option of recording the entire interaction. This solution allows doctors to conduct highly critical diagnostics such as Diacom viewing and detection of Thrombolysis in cardiac care. The CISCO's Virtual Expertise Digital

Solution is encrypted to protect the patient related information. It ensures that there will be no leakage of information during its storage and transmission while using the solution.

Under the agreement, Narayana Health and CISCO decided to work together in setting up advanced telemedicine solutions across 3 centers in India – Sirsi and Bellary in Karnataka, and Rajarhat in Bengal via the main centre at Narayana Health City located in Bommasandra, Bangalore, Karnataka.

Sankara Nethralaya

Ophthalmology lends itself easily to telemedicine as it is largely image based diagnosis. Sankara Nethralaya offers tele ophthalmology services to rural areas. The services include comprehensive eye examination, training school teachers for vision screening programs, organizing diabetic retinopathy screening camps and performing eye surgeries free of cost at the base hospital.

Scope of Telemedicine in Rural India

Public Private Partnership is required to make telemedicine a success in India.

It is important that before entering a rural market, a thorough analysis of the local medical system prevalent there, should be done. Companies providing telemedicine healthcare services should collaborate with other such providers so that they together mount some pressure on the government for extending its support and provides financial assistance to the private players.

Many private companies don't see Indian rural areas as potential markets for providing telemedicine services. Since profit is limited in serving rural areas, companies that provide healthcare services need alternate profit streams.

In villages, inferior quality medicines are supplied by the chemists of the local drug stores. Also limited and only common types of drugs are available in such stores. The healthcare providing companies can make profit by opening their own drug shops where a wide range of quality medicines should be made available.

In many rural areas, the quality of water available for drinking is very poor. So in such areas, the demand for clean drinking water can be met by the healthcare providing companies. To earn profits, they can open a chain that provides portable drinking water cans at reasonable price to households in those areas.

In rural areas, training centers should be established to give training to local people regarding the use of different equipments that form part of telemedicine set up. Such training centers are beneficial for both the healthcare providing companies as well as for rural population. On the one hand companies can make profits by establishing such centers and on the other hand, these centers open employment opportunities for the trainees.

Technological Paradigm Shift

When the first telemedicine pilot project was started in India, satellite was used to establish links between peripheral healthcare centers and referral hospitals. At that time cellular network for mobile communication as well as optical fiber network for internet communication was not fully developed and distributed across the country. But times have changed now, with the expansion of cellular and optical fiber networks throughout the nation, the accessibility to mobile and internet services have increased many folds even in rural areas. Internet and mobiles can enhance the effectiveness and range of telemedicine services by allowing faster transmission of large data files at relatively lower costs. Earlier video conferencing which is the crux of telemedicine in India was possible only through the satellites but now video conferencing can be easily done through internet or even through mobiles. In such a scenario, technology shift is very important. The old telemedicine infrastructure needs to be replaced by new one which should be compatible with the recent mobile and internet technologies.

Conclusion

It is true that telemedicine is not a substitute for traditional healthcare system, but it is surely helpful in bridging disparity in quality and access to healthcare between urban and rural areas of India. Telemedicine is successful in providing basic healthcare services at affordable price to the underserved population of India.

References

1. Ebad, R. (Nov, 2013). Telemedicine: Current and Future Perspectives. *International Journal of Computer Science Issues, 10(6),* 242-49.

2. Bhowmik, D., Duraivel, S., Singh, R.K. et al. (2013). Telemedicine- An Innovating Healthcare System in India. *The Pharma Innovation Journal, 2(4),* 1-20.

3. Mishra, S.K., Kapoor, L., & Singh, I.P. (July/Aug, 2009). Telemedicine in India: Current Scenario and the Future. *Telemedicine and e Health,* 568-76.

4. O' Connell, P. (2015). Advantages and Challenges to using Telehealth Medicine. *Global Journal of Medical Research: F Diseases, 15(4),* 19-22.

5. Garg, V., Brewer, J. (May, 2011). Telemedicine Security: A Systematic Review. *Journal of Diabetes Science and Technology, 5(3),* 768-77.

6. Ganpathy, K. (2006). Telemedicine in India. *ABPN, 10(19),* 1086-91.

7. Dasgupta, A, Soumya, D. (Jan, 2008). Telemedicine: A New Horizon in Public Health in India. *Indian Journal of Community Medicine, 33(1),* 3-8.

8. Rajaguru, H., Prabhakar, S.K. (2017). Development of an Efficient Epilepsy Classification System from ECG Signals for Telemedicine Application. *International Journal of Civil Engineering and Technology, 8(12),* 38-52.

9. Saravann, S. (2012). Internet Based Mobile Telemedicine Using Computer Communication Network. *International Journal of Computer Engineering and Technology, 3(2)*, 213-31.

10. Mehta, K.G., Chavda, P. (2013). Telemedicine: A boon and the Promise to Rural India. *J Rev Prog*, 1-3.

11. Kumar, A., Ahmad, S. (2015). A Review Study on Utilization of Telemedicine and e-Health Services in Public Health. *Asian Pac J Health Sci*, 60-68.

MCQs

1. Which of the following is not the characteristic of Asynchronous type technology?

a) This technology is also called 'store and forward'.

b) Digital camera is used to take digital images which are stored and then forwarded to another location by a computer.

c) In this technology real time data is exchanged.

d) None of the above

2. Who started the first telemedicine pilot project in India in the year 2001?

a) World Health Partners

b) Narayana Health

c) Sankara Nethralaya

d) ISRO in collaboration with Apollo Hospitals Group

3. What is the advantage of telemedicine?

a) It improves access to quality health services for the population living in underserved areas.

b) It eliminates distance barriers.

c) It is helpful in critical care situations where moving a patient is undesirable or not feasible.

d) All of the above

4. **Which of the following North Eastern States of India has set an example of successful implementation of telemedicine program in the country?**

   a) Assam

   b) Tripura

   c) Arunachal Pradesh

   d) Meghalaya

5. **In which year the Ministry of Health and Family Welfare, GOI defined National Standards on telemedicine?**

   a) 2001

   b) 2003

   c) 2007

   d) 2013

6. **In which year the Ministry of Health and Family Welfare, GOI established National Rural Telemedicine Network?**

   a) 2007

   b) 2008

   c) 2009

   d) 2010

7. **In which Five Year Plan, the Ministry of Health and Family Welfare, GOI introduced m-Health which involves use of mobile phones to speed up transmission?**

   a) 11th Five Year Plan

   b) 10th Five Year Plan

   c) 12th Five Year Plan

   d) None of the above

8. **In which year the Ministry of Health and Family Welfare, GOI launched a telemedicine service named 'Sehat' through which people in rural areas can consult doctors through video link and can also online order generic drugs?**

    a) 2012

    b) 2013

    c) 2015

    d) 2016

9. **Apollo Telemedicine Networking Foundation uses which of the following web enabled Telemedicine Application?**

    a) Medintegra WEB

    b) ALTHEA

    c) CISCO's Virtual Expertise Digital Solution

    d) None of the above

10. **Under which Apollo Hospital's initiative, Tele health services are provided on mobile phones and tablets?**

    a) New Age Telemedicine

    b) m Telemedicine

    c) Telemedicine 2.0

    d) None of the above

11. **Which of the following digital solutions is generally used by WHP coordinated 'sky centers'?**

    a) CISCO's Virtual Expertise Digital Solution

    b) ALTHEA

    c) eClinicalWorks

    d) athenahealth

12. Which of the following digital solutions is generally used by Narayana Health to deliver affordable healthcare services remotely?

a) CISCO's Virtual Expertise Digital Solution

b) EpicCare Ambulatory

c) eClinicalWorks

d) ALTHEA

Answer key

1. (c)   2. (d)   3. (d)   4. (b)   5. (b)   6. (a)   7. (c)   8. (c)

9. (a)   10. (c)   11. (b)   12. (a)

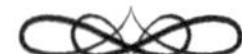

Chapter 6

Importance of Patient Experience in Healthcare Planning

Abstract

Patient experience is an important indicator to measure the quality of care provided by healthcare organizations. This chapter gives an insight into patient experience framework and its facets, relevance of patient engagement, role of technology in measuring patient satisfaction, health insurance issues and ways to improve patient experience.

Introduction

In today's culture of healthcare, patient experience is fast getting in the spotlight.

A patient's experience starts as soon as he/she enters a hospital. The hospital environment; waiting time; interaction with physician, nursing and other paramedical staff; quality of treatment given; lab and pharmacy services; discharge information, all these factors contribute to patient experience. If a patient is satisfied with all of these things, then he/she will have a good experience in the hospital.

One of the important aspects of patient experience is the patient's perception of the varied interactions that he/she has across the episode or continuum of care.

For a good patient experience, it is important that interaction between the physician and patient is more effective. This can be achieved by having an empathetic attitude towards patients, by listening to them carefully and by encouraging them to indulge in self care.

Patient Experience Framework

Following are the few facets of patient experience framework-

1. Respect patient's preferences and care needs. This may include cultural, religious and social needs.

2. Provide coordinated care across health and social care system to ensure seamless care delivery.

3. Protect patient's right to privacy of his/her healthcare information. The patient reserves the right to share it if he/she so desires.

4. Provide information to the patients regarding their health status, progress, laboratory tests and prognosis to keep them updated and make them self reliant to take their own decisions.

5. Give emotional support to take care of patient's anxiety and fear in case of chronic diseases like cancer.

6. Ensure an easy and seamless access to care.

7. Maintain patient's uninterrupted care continuum across multiple care settings such as hospital, home and community.

8. Involve family and friends as care givers. These people play an important role in patient's care especially when the patient is cognitively challenged.

Patient Centered Approach

In patient centered approach, patient is not just a passive recipient but an active partner in his/her care with a right to make decisions regarding his/her treatment options. The patient is provided with necessary information so that he/she can take decisions.

Patient Consumerism

Treating patient as a consumer has the following advantages-

1. Shared decision making.

2. Involvement in wellness and preventive care programs.

3. Awareness of one's own health.

The consumerism of patient care has an impact on patient experience.

But some of the physicians feel that patient consumerism is likely to affect the relationship that the doctors have with their patients. They believe that, through patient consumerism, healthcare may transform into a commodity.

According to physicians, some of the disadvantages associated with treating a patient as consumer are-

1. Disruption of trust between physicians and patients.

2. Rise of illegal means of delivering services like paying physicians under the table to receive better care.

Following points should be considered while treating a patient as a consumer-

1. Level of healthcare literacy

2. Access to care and services

3. Healthcare financing options

Stakeholders in Healthcare

For a good patient experience, identification and involvement of stakeholders is important. It is the responsibility of the stakeholders to take right decision for patients.

In healthcare, primary stakeholders include patients, their immediate and extended family members; physician and his/her team (that includes primary care physicians, surgeons, radiologists, specialists etc.); hospital staff (nurses, therapists, laboratory personnel, pharmacists, dietitians, medical records departmental staff, other paramedical staff etc.); health insurance payers, employers etc. Secondary stakeholders include government and regulatory agencies, disease management organizations, health information technology organizations, health and wellness organizations, medical schools etc.

Voice of Customer (VOC)

In a hospital scenario, voice of the customer (VOC) is captured by taking patients' feedback to determine their satisfaction level and their expectations. The patient's feedback can be taken through different ways like-

(i) Surveys

(ii) Customer complaint databases.

(iii) Management rounds and interaction with patients.

VOC helps the managers of a healthcare organization in the following processes-

(i) Identifying and prioritizing patient's needs and concerns.

(ii) Creating new service lines and models of care.

(iii) Customizing the service based on preferences of the patients.

Healthcare Marketing

Marketing in healthcare is a new concept. Care delivery centers opt for marketing their patient centric services so that patients can choose from varied services they offer.

Patient markets span a variety of promotional approaches that include disease awareness advertising, branded promotion of products, condition management support advertising etc.

Niche marketing concept advocates marketing for a niche group of patients such as cancer care, chronic care, emergency care etc.

Marketing of healthcare services commonly done through

(i) Social media

(ii) External marketing agencies

(iii) Newspapers and health magazines

Patient Expectations

During the hospital stay, a patient wants to be kept well informed about his/her health. He/she wants to be involved in his/her care related decisions. He/she needs attention of the staff and expects the staff to be sensitive and polite. All these factors contribute to patient's satisfaction.

Patients and their family members look for a few of the following when they seek healthcare services-

(i) Reasonable waiting time

(ii) Value for money

(iii) Friendly staff

In United States, the Affordable Care Act associates performance related to patient experience metrics to reimbursement. For hospitals, it is an important driver for improving patient experience.

Cultural Factors

In India, cultural factors play an important role in defining patient experience, e.g. some patients may be sensitive about auspicious timings, some may have preferences with respect to diet, some may prefer to be treated with a physician belonging to a particular ethnicity etc.

The healthcare providers should pay attention towards these cultural factors because they have a critical impact on patient experience.

Role of Leadership

Leadership of a healthcare organization has significant role in ensuring that the patients have good experience in hospital settings. Patient centered care has to be a strategic priority for the leaders. Leaders who encourage risk, open to new ideas and actively seek feedback from staff are able to develop better patient centered care models. While developing healthcare policies, superior quality of care provided in an affordable, effective and safe way with the best possible patient experience should be the aim of leaders.

Hospitality in Healthcare

Hospitals consider hospitality as a major part of their progress in this competitive world. Hospitality is integrated with healthcare to provide unique experience to the patients.

Hospitals are now seen as a place of comfort care with best modern facilities along with prevention, diagnosis, treatment and cure of diseases.

Following are the factors that are part of hospitality management in hospitals-

1. Amenities- It includes food, private rooms, cable TV, Wi-Fi etc.

2. Nursing- Attentiveness, responsiveness and courtesy shown by nursing staff.

3. Treatment and therapies- It includes pain management, stress management, meditation area, vaccination and immunization facilities.

4. Security- It comprises patient safety and privacy, security alarms and security guards.

5. Physicians and staff- Access to physicians; empathy, sound knowledge, attentiveness and compassion shown by physicians and other staff.

6. Hospital Environment- Cleanliness, sanitation, hygiene, comfortable and relaxing environment.

7. Admission and discharge- Hospital management information system, computer connectivity, timely discharge, follow up, information desk and support facilities.

8. Other facilities- ATMs, cafeteria etc.

Dietary services are the crucial part of hospitality in hospitals. Most of the corporate hospitals recruit professionals from the hospitality background to ensure that patient satisfaction, convenience and quality standards must be maintained while serving therapeutic diet to the patients. The types of diet serve to patients include normal diet, liquid diet, low salt based diet, diabetic diet, low fat diet, high fiber diet, semi-solid diet, soft diet, high protein diet, Ryle's tube diet etc.

Dieticians plan the meal for patients on a case to case basis. It involves identifying what needs to be served to the patients, in what quantity and at what time.

Hospitals provide balanced and hygienic therapeutic diet to patients. Its purpose is to maintain good nutritional status, to correct deficiencies, to prevent a number of diseases and to maintain body's ability to metabolize the nutrients. Overall dieticians help in developing, strengthening and implementing some effective health policies to improve diet and encourage the regular practice of keeping good health.

Sanitation and cleanliness are other important aspects of healthcare hospitality. Hospitals have become extra cautious and housekeeping has become an essential part of hospitality. In the corporate hospitals, for the comfort of visitors and relatives of patients, there are spacious waiting areas with comfortable reclining chairs and couches. People come to hospital for various reasons. Some experiences are joyful like the birth of a child and some are sorrowful like casualties, diseases, deaths. It is the responsibility of the hospital to make patients feel comfortable in every situation. The hospital staff should make it a priority to provide quality treatment to patients so that they can recover quickly and get discharged as soon as possible. The patients need to be fully attended during their entire stay at the hospital. The staff should also ensure their smooth discharge from the hospital. These days, people prefer the use of debit and credit cards, net banking and mobile banking facilities. All these facilities should be available in hospitals for the convenience of patients. To encourage medical tourism, modern hospitals provide facilities like foreign currency conversion counters, interpreter of languages, transportation means etc.

Continuous Quality Improvement (CQI)

It is a quality process that encompasses monitoring and improving performance of patient care on an ongoing basis. It is important for healthcare organizations to have a CQI strategy in order to deliver high performance. Measuring and improving care delivery and service operations from the patient's perspective to deliver a superior patient experience has become one of the top priorities of the healthcare systems.

Following are the few CQI approaches-

1. Lean CQI strategy – It focuses on streamlining processes at all levels of care.

2. Six sigma – It focuses on removing sources of error.

3. PDCA cycle – It has the following steps

   (i) Plan – Seek an opportunity for improvement and plan a change.

   (ii) Do – Implement the change.

   (iii) Check – Determine the effectiveness of change by analyzing data.

   (iv) Act – If the change is effective, implement it on a larger scale. If not, start the cycle again.

Gathering data on an ongoing basis and continuously monitoring the outcome of interventions are crucial for CQI. Management can work on gaps that are found to make necessary changes. It is important not only to implement interventions to improve the patient experience, but also to ensure that they remain effective. Monitoring these interventions in real time, helps create a better experience for the patients.

Satisfaction Survey

Healthcare satisfaction survey is a valuable tool to improve operational performance. The healthcare satisfaction survey captures the voice of patients and their care givers, staff such as physicians, nurses etc.

The data obtained through these surveys is helpful in-

   (i) Diagnosing organizational problems

   (ii) Developing initiatives

   (iii) Implementing plans for organizational changes

   (iv) Monitoring changes and interventions

Patient Engagement

Research has proven that along with healthcare professionals, patient's engagement in his/her own health and decision making results in improved health outcomes. Patient experience is a function of patient engagement. The more inclusive the patient engagement, the more is the patient satisfaction.

Information technology helps healthcare providers in supporting patient engagement initiative.

Healthcare Information Management Systems Society provides a 5 stages roadmap for patient education.

(i) Inform me

(ii) Engage me

(iii) Empower me

(iv) Partner with me

(v) Support my e-community

While the healthcare professionals look to engage patients in their own care, the onus of cooperating with them lies on the patient. It is important that the patient be a manager of his/her own care and be involved in it on a day to day basis in order to take timely decisions and manage risks related to diagnosis or treatment options.

Self management can be in two forms-

(i) Patient provider partnership – It involves patients in a collaborative care.

(ii) Self management education – It involves learning technical skills and problem solving skills.

Key concept in both the above approaches is the ability to make patient self reliant and drive in him/her the confidence to carry out actions in favour of his/her goals. Self efficacy helps in minimizing costs and improving health outcomes.

Benefits of Patient Engagement

1. Increased patient satisfaction – Patient himself/herself is involved in his/her care so there is a sense of satisfaction.

2. Reduced costs – Timely care and actions minimize patient's hospitalization rate. Self education and self help measures avoid costs.

3. Timely care – Since the patient is aware of the complications, he/she can take necessary actions on time.

4. Community benefits – Patient is a part of community and patient education goes a long way in helping communities stay healthy.

Following are the number of factors that need to be overcome to carry out effective patient engagement-

1. **Health literacy** – Low health literacy leads to poor patient engagement.

2. **Cultural diversity** – Patient's degree of engagement is affected by cultural differences and other factors like age, gender, education level, socio-economic status, religious beliefs etc. To overcome these factors, an adequate degree of sensitivity is required on the part of healthcare providers so that they are able to engage patients more effectively.

3. **Behavioural and cognitive impairment**– These limitations can be overcome by involving other stakeholders in decision making and present the things in simpler form to help patients understand them easily.

4. **Financial considerations** – Generally patients want less costly treatment. This may go against the care they need. It is important to guide the patients on treatment choices and their related costs.

Following are the few patient engagement methodologies-

1. Passive Patient Education

In this, text based on audio-visual patient education material is delivered to the patient by a healthcare professional. Patients read and practice the activities as desired. This method requires minimum additional costs and resources. Here the involvement of patient is minimal to moderate.

2. Active Information

In this, healthcare centers/professionals with the help of information technology send prompts to the patients that guide them to take an action. It is a cost intensive model. Some institutes may not have the necessary infrastructure to support it. Here the patient involvement is moderate to high.

3. Active information along with patient collaboration

In this, tools are focused on supporting, creating and maintaining collaboration with the patient during his/her hospital visit or stay. It is designed for multiple points of engagement. It supports activities like disease management seminars, enrolling patients in transition care plans, medication guidance and chronic care support. This model is feasible for those institutes where both human and material resources are available. It is also cost intensive. Here the patient involvement is very high.

Health Coaching

Health coaching is defined as helping patients gain knowledge, skills and techniques to become active participants in their own care. It leads to better health outcomes. Coaching is imparted to provide health information, to teach disease specific and problem solving skills and to promote healthy behaviour. Coaches can help patients cope with negative emotions during the treatment for chronic diseases. This helps in improving patient experience. Health coaching can be helpful in understanding the need of continuity of care.

Following are the models of coaching-

1. Teamlet Model

In a teamlet model, a health coach (a nurse or health practitioner) is paired with the physician and imparts information to the patient relevant to his/her condition after the physician's assessment.

2. Care Coordinator Model

In this model, a care coordinator is assigned to the patient who helps him/her with transitions of care and follow ups. It also involves homecare visits.

Technology in Healthcare

Technology has revolutionized our way of living and its presence is felt and needed in every aspect of life. It has found its application in healthcare as well. The various applications of technology in healthcare include electronic medical records, medical devices, technology enabled services like telemedicine etc.

Social Media

Social media is changing the way patients and healthcare providers interact. According to a survey, approximately 90% of 18-24 years old respondents indicated that they would engage in health activities through social media. Approximately 50% of respondents expected their healthcare providers to respond within a few hours to appointment requests made via social media. It was observed that people spent more time on healthcare consumer community sites than the healthcare community sites.

mHealth

mHealth is a component of eHealth. According to Global Observatory for eHealth, mHealth is defined as medical and public health practice supported by mobile devices such as mobile phones, patient monitoring devices, personal digital assistant and other wireless devices.

Following are the applications of mobile technology-

1. Healthcare call centre services and emergency toll free telephone services.

2. Mobile telemedicine

3. Appointment scheduling and reminder services, health promotion initiatives.

4. Medical record keeping

Information technology helps healthcare organizations in the following ways-

1. Information Gathering

Effective early intervention may require timely access to large quantities of information. IT enabled services have a potential to gather a large amount of information directly through people. Social networking sites where patients interact are means of getting the voice of client. Medical data in personal health records, electronic health records is useful when pooled at a central place for decision making.

2. Information Integration

It is important to integrate the information at one place and decipher its meaning to take necessary actions.

3. Information Management

Healthcare organizations develop databases to organize and analyze the information gathered. This enables analysts to develop innovative intervention and engagement strategies.

4. Information Analysis

The analysts work on the information captured and note new patterns and trends that are emerging.

Barriers in Communication

Poor literacy or language skills can become a major hindrance in communication between patients and healthcare providers. Lack of communication results in-

(i) Lower and inadequate use of wellness and preventive care services by the patients.

(ii) Misdiagnosis or delayed diagnosis

(iii) Increased hospital admissions and readmissions

(iv) Adverse effects of medication due to inability to understand prescription.

Hospitals and other care settings such as community clinics, psychiatric facilities, nursing facilities etc. ease communication by using IT enabled bilingual translators and interpreters.

Telemedicine

In a resource poor setting where there is a difficulty in providing primary care, technologies such as telemedicine is considered to be a boon.

Following are the advantages of telemedicine-

(i) Patients from remote areas can more easily obtain clinical services through telemedicine.

(ii) With the help of telemedicine, hospitals can provide emergency and intensive care services to remote and inaccessible areas.

(iii) Specialists can serve more patients using telemedicine technologies in areas where there is a shortage of medical professionals.

(iv) Telemedicine improves patients' engagement as they can stay in their local communities and when hospitalized away from home, can keep in contact with family and friends.

Measuring Patient Satisfaction

Across the world there is an increasing emphasis on measuring patient satisfaction to assess the quality of services. Although it has some inherent flaws, measuring patient experience has become a vital part of continuous quality improvement strategy for the hospitals. The information must be collected from multiple sources by using a variety of methods to get a clear picture of patient's level of satisfaction.

Several market research studies have reported that only a small percentage of dissatisfied customers complain to the service provider, and about 96% tell nine to ten of their friends about unpleasant experience. This grapevine effect can become even more powerful when consumers take advantage of the internet to voice their complaints. Many internet sites have inbuilt software to allow patients to evaluate and assess their experiences with a hospital, doctor, service group or insurance and other medical plans online and some have the capacity to include written comments. Many service providers publish ratings of patient experience as part of their online directories. It is necessary for the patient focused organizations to handle the unhappy patients effectively by addressing their concerns in order to create a reputation that the service providers value patients.

Service Recovery

Service recovery is defined as the process to recover dissatisfied or lost customers or patients by identifying, analyzing and fixing the problem.

Good service recovery program is an effective tool for improving level of patient satisfaction.

Service recovery can be done in the following ways-

1. Apologize/acknowledge
2. Listen, emphasize and ask open questions
3. Fix the problem quickly and fairly
4. Offer atonement
5. Follow up
6. Remember your promise

Good service recovery programs look for long term solutions and go beyond the quick fix. They include a process of tracking problems and complaints to identify the source of problem so that right intervention can be put into place.

When management implements recovery programs, it is important to differentiate between the 'strategic initiatives' that should be in place before the actual problem occurs and the 'tactical activities' that should happen after a problem has occurred.

Health Insurance

Healthcare industry in India is in a state of significant transition due to various factors like health consciousness among various sections of society, price liberalization, reduction in bureaucracy, increasing awareness, introduction of private healthcare financing etc.

Various health insurance products available in the country and the insurance schemes can be broadly categorized as-

1. Voluntary health insurance schemes or private for profit schemes.

2. Mandatory health insurance schemes or government run schemes.

3. Insurance offered by NGOs/community based health insurance.

4. Employee based schemes.

In private for profit insurance, buyers are willing to pay premium to an insurance company that groups similar risks and insures for health related expenses. The main distinction between private for profit scheme and others is that the former sets premiums at a level which is based on assessment of risk status of a customer and accordingly the level of risk mitigation is provided rather than as a linkage to a proportion of customer's income.

The privatization improves the performance of insurance sector in India which leads to better patient satisfaction. But the critics of private insurance argue that privatization diverts scarce resources away from the poor, enhances health costs, allows cream skimming. [Cream skimming is a practice where the insurers selectively insure those who are healthy with less risk of falling ill to increase the profits]. According to the critics, private health insurance ignores the social aspect of health protection. In contrast, supporters of private health insurance believe that private insurance bridges financing gaps by offering consumers higher value for money and help them avoid long waiting time, low quality care and under the table payments. These problems are faced by those who use public health facilities for free or participate in mandatory social insurance schemes.

As health insurance sector in India is still in its nascent phase, the role of Insurance Regulatory and Development Authority (IRDA) is very crucial. It has to assure that this sector grows rapidly and the benefits of insurance go to the consumers by guarding them against the ill effects of insurance privatization. Privatization and development related to health insurance need to be managed properly otherwise it may have negative impact on healthcare primarily to the large segment of rural population of India. A well managed insurance sector can improve access to care and health status of people in a country significantly. If the privatization of health insurance is not properly regulated, it can have adverse effect on the cost of patient care, health equity and patient satisfaction. Therefore it is the responsibility of IRDA to protect the interests of policy holders, to promote efficiency in insurance business, to regulate prices and to review terms and conditions of policies.

Managing Patient Experience

Hospitals can minimize the incidents of poor service by implementing an effective patient feedback mechanism that encourages the patients to report.

Following are the potential clinical and operational risks linked to poor patient experience-

1. Clinical Risks

    (i) Reduced patient cooperation in prevention practices.

    (ii) Reduced patient compliance with disease management.

    (iii) Reduced patient compliance with advice and treatment regimes.

2. Operational Risks

(i) Impact on satisfaction, attentiveness and attendance of staff and increased staff turnover.

(ii) Poor communication between patients and healthcare professionals.

(iii) Dissatisfied patients can be more costly to handle, they make more demands   and exhibit less cooperation and patience.

Each of the above risks contributes to increased cost of patient care and may lead to reduced success in achieving optimum clinical outcomes.

Following are the few important steps to be considered while collecting information on patient experience-

1. Don't just depend upon annual satisfaction surveys but use multiple methods (formal, informal) to collect the information.

2. Triangulate quantitative (numbers) and qualitative (stories, narrations) data.

3. Give equal importance to compliments and complaints.

Data should:

1. Be in real time, collected regularly and systematically by using appropriate tools and technologies.

2. Be direct and relevant as much as possible for specific services.

3. Be collected for both along care pathways and also for single episode of care.

4. Allow for comparisons over time, within and between services and organizations.

5. Focus on patient's and service user's feelings and emotions about the way they are treated, as well as on actual story behind the incidents happened.

6. Put patients at centre by selectively measuring what matters to patients.

Use Patient Feedback to improve services:

1. Explicitly promote the strategy of improving patient experience across the teams.

2. Develop and support the expertise in managing patient experience among the teams.

3. Make improvement of patient experience a necessary part of all quality improvement programs.

Facilitate and support the ongoing involvement of patients:

1. Data collection process should involve patients and staff where staff gets an opportunity to hear directly from patients.

2. Staff and patients can work together on projects to co-design/co-produce existing or new services.

3. Include marginalized/under privileged patients whose voice is not heard.

4. Keep patients informed about the various steps after data collection like analysis results etc.

Prepare the staff and equip them to respond:

1. Give feedback to staff about patient experience.

2. Staff development programs should proactively include a session on improving patient experience.

To get full picture, triangulate data from different sources such as:

1. Patient stories including anecdotes

2. Surveys

3. Specific feedback and complaints

4. Incident reports

5. General feedback

6. Media reports

Following is the critical list of actions for management to improve patient experience-

1. At the strategic level, managers need to frame patient experience as an integral and equal part of the quality framework, alongside clinical effectiveness and safety.

2. Ensure that the board receives regular and meaningful reports on patient experience.

3. Recognize the link between patient experience and staff well-being and develop plans for improving both.

4. Support and encourage leaders at all levels to create an organizational culture that prioritizes work on understanding and improving experiences of patients.

5. Build and articulate carefully the business case for investing in the measurement and improvement of patient experience.

6. Make focus on delivering a positive patient experience an essential part of staff induction, development and appraisal.

7. Make understanding and improving patient experience a vital part of in-house leadership development programs (including for middle managers and clinicians).

Conclusion

It can be concluded that improving patient experience in healthcare organizations can lead to higher quality care, more satisfied staff, fewer preventable medical errors, fewer malpractice law suits and an improved financial bottom line.

References

1. Carroll, P. (2012). *Patient Satisfaction- Understanding and Managing the Experience of Care.* Irwin Press.

2. Mosadeghrad, A.M. (2014). Factors Influencing Healthcare Service Quality. *International Journal of Health Policy and Management, 3(2),* 77.

3. Zeithaml, V., Bitner, M.J., & Gremler D.D. (2013). *Services Marketing: Integrating Customer Focus across the Firm (6ᵗʰ edition)*. New York: Mc Graw Hill.

4. Bhat, R. (2005). *Third Party Administrators and Health Insurance in India: Perception of Providers and Policy Holders.*

5. Bawa, S.K., & Verma, R. (2011). Third Party Administrators (TPAs) in India: An Insight into Role Defined and Role Played with Reference to IRDA. *Zenith International Journal of Multidisciplinary Research, 3.*

6. Cleary, P.D. (2016). Evolving Concepts of Patient Centered Care and the Assessment of Patient Care Experiences: Optimism and Opposition. *Journal of Health Politics, Policy and Law, 41(4),* 675-96.

7. Anhang, P.R., Elliott, M.N. et al. (July, 2014). Examining the Role of Patient Experience Surveys in Measuring Health Care Quality. *Medical Care Research and Review, 71(5),* 522-54.

8. Ahmed, F., Burt, J., & Roland, M. (2014). Measuring Patient Experience: Concepts and Methods. *Patient, 7,* 235-41.

9. Fredericks, S., Lapum, J., & Hui, G. (2015). Examining the Effect of Patient Centered Care on Outcomes. *Br. J. Nurs, 24,* 394-400.

10. Legg, A., Andrews, S., & Huynh, H. et al. (2014). Patient's Anxiety and Hope: Predictors and Adherence Intensions in an Acute Care Context. *Health Expect, 18,* 3034-43.

MCQs

1. Which of the following factors does not contribute to the patient experience?

a) Waiting time

b) Quality of treatment given

c) Source of hospital funding

d) Interaction with physician, nursing and other paramedical staff.

2. How can physician and patient interaction become more effective?

    a) By having an empathetic attitude towards patients.

    b) By encouraging them to indulge in self care.

    c) By listening to them carefully.

    d) All of the above

3. Which of the following is not a characteristic of patient centered approach?

    a) Patient has a right to make decisions regarding his/her treatment options.

    b) Patient is a passive recipient of healthcare.

    c) Patient is provided with necessary information so that he/she can take decisions.

    d) None of the above

4. Which of the following is not an advantage of treating patient as a consumer?

    a) Rise of illegal means of delivering services like paying physicians under the table to receive better care.

    b) Awareness of one's own health.

    c) Shared decision making.

    d) Involvement in wellness and preventive care programs.

5. Which among the following are the secondary stakeholders in healthcare?

    a) Physician and his/her team

    b) Hospital staff

    c) Government and regulatory agencies

    d) Health insurance payers

6. **Which of the following is not the way of taking patient's feedback?**

    a) Surveys

    b) Management rounds and interaction with patients.

    c) Customer complaint databases

    d) Asking doctors about the patient's feedback.

7. **Marketing of healthcare services is done through:**

    a) Social media

    b) Newspapers and health magazines

    c) Both (a) and (b)

    d) None of the above

8. **Which country introduces 'Affordable Care Act' that associates performance related to patient experience metrics to reimbursement?**

    a) India

    b) Germany

    c) China

    d) United States

9. **What is the quality that helps healthcare leaders to develop better patient centered care models?**

    a) Discourage risks

    b) Actively seek feedback from staff.

    c) Both (a) and (b)

    d) None of the above

10. Which of the following is not the purpose of providing therapeutic diet to patients in hospitals?

a) To maintain the body's ability to metabolize nutrients.

b) To correct deficiencies.

c) To satisfy the taste buds of patients.

d) To maintain good nutritional status.

11. Which of the following CQI approaches focuses on removing sources of error?

a) Lean CQI strategy

b) PDCA cycle

c) Six sigma

d) None of the above

12. Which of the following is not the benefit of patient engagement?

a) Increased patient satisfaction

b) Increased costs

c) Timely care

d) Community benefits

13. Which of the following is not the characteristic of 'Passive Patient Education' patient engagement methodology?

a) Involvement of patient is maximum

b) Text based on audio-visual patient education is delivered to the patient by a healthcare professional.

c) Minimum additional costs and resources are required.

d) Patients read and practice the activities as desired.

14. **Which of the following is not the characteristic of 'Active information along with patient collaboration' patient engagement methodology?**

    a) It is designed for multiple points of engagement.

    b) It is feasible for those institutes where both human and material resources are available.

    c) It is a low cost model.

    d) Here patient involvement is very high.

15. **Which of the following is defined as helping patients gain knowledge, skills and techniques to become active participants in their own care?**

    a) Healthcare Marketing

    b) Health Coaching

    c) Health Insurance

    d) None of the above

16. **Which of the following is defined as medical and public health practice supported by mobile devices such as mobile phones, personal digital assistant and other wireless devices?**

    a) Digital Health

    b) mHealth

    c) eHealth

    d) None of the above

17. **Which of the following statements is false regarding telemedicine?**

    a) Specialists can serve fewer patients using telemedicine technologies in areas where there is a shortage of medical professionals.

    b) Patients from remote areas can more easily obtain clinical services through telemedicine.

    c) With the help of telemedicine, hospitals can provide emergency and intensive care services to remote and inaccessible areas.

d) Telemedicine improves patients' engagement as they can stay in their local communities and when hospitalized away from home, can keep in contact with family and friends.

18. How can service recovery in healthcare be defined?

a) It is the process of recovering dissatisfied or lost customers or patients by identifying, analyzing and fixing the problem.

b) It is the process of recovering losses suffered by a healthcare organization by increasing the patient's bill.

c) It is the process of reintroducing the service provided by a healthcare organization which it has earlier stopped.

d) None of the above

19. Which of the following insurance schemes sets premiums at a level which is based on assessment of risk status of a customer and accordingly the level of risk mitigation is provided?

a) Government run schemes

b) Insurance offered by NGOs

c) Private for profit schemes

d) None of the above

20. Which of the following statements is false about private health insurance scheme?

a) It allows cream skimming.

b) It diverts scarce resources away from the poor.

c) It enhances health costs.

d) It leads to low quality care.

21. Which among the following is not a clinical risk associated with poor patient experience?

a) Increased staff turnover.

b) Reduced patient compliance with disease management.

c) Reduced patient compliance with advice and treatment regimes.

d) Reduced patient cooperation in prevention practices.

Answer key

1. (c)	2. (d)	3. (b)	4. (a)	5. (c)	6. (d)	7. (c)	8. (d)
9. (b)	10. (c)	11. (c)	12. (b)	13. (a)	14. (c)	15. (b)	16. (b)
17. (a)	18. (a)	19. (c)	20. (d)	21. (a)			

Index

A

D

E

M

Malicious Users   98

Malvertising   101

Managerial Indicators   74

Managing Patient Experience   143

Mandatory Health Insurance   6

Measuring Patient Satisfaction   141

Medical Asepsis   69

Medicare   2, 5, 9

Medicare Benefits Scheme   9

Medication error   65

Medintegra WEB   118

mHealth   138

N

Narayana Health   119

National

   Accreditation Board for Hospitals and Healthcare Providers   60

   Exit Test   61

   Health Service   13

   Institute of Health   2

O

P

Q

R

S

T